INTRODUCTION

Evidence from looking at pictures of Americans taken at turn of the 20th century then compared to those taken 100-years later shows the effect of diet on our appearance. The early 1900-photos show virtually no obese people; even the elderly have flat stomachs with no excess fat showing. But today, roughly 1/3rd of us are carrying way-too much body fat. Between 1890 and 2000, the prevalence of obesity increased from 3.4% to 35%.[1] Overeating and poor food choices are the culprits. Americans in 1900 consumed 90% of their calories from whole plant foods with the remnant from animal sources (meats, dairy, fish). In 2000, the opposite resulted, 90% calories came from animal foods but only 10% from plant food sources. It is interesting to note that the leading causes of death in 1900 were also very different than those reported in 1997: [2]

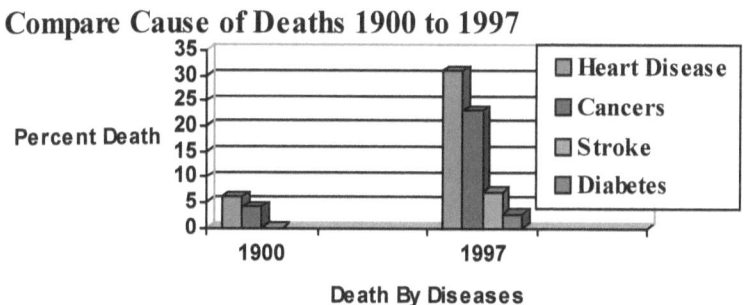

Compare Cause of Deaths 1900 to 1997

[1] Helmchen LA, Henderson RM. Changes in the distribution of body mass index ofwhite US men, 1890-2000. Ann Hum Biol. 2004 Mar-Apr;31(2):174-81.
[2] Source: 1900-1970, U.S. Public Health Service, Vital Statistics of the United States, annual, Vol. I and Vol II; 1971-2001, U.S. National Center for Health Statistics, Vital Statistics of the United States, annual; National Vital Statistics Report (NVSR) (formerly Monthly Vital Statistics Report); and unpublished data.

Humans are eating foods that may be the cause of diseases. A great deal of evidence identifies the mechanism with our increased love affair with animal foods. The antithesis that eating a whole plant food menu prevents or reverses diseases attributed to animal-foods is well supported. Simply out, American preference for 90% of their calories from whole plant foods in 1900 restrained both heart disease and cancer death rates to 6% or less. Then a century later, when America adopted eating mostly animal source foods, heart disease increased 575% and cancers increased 516%! Food choice is the culprit associated with compromised health issues resulting in diseases.

When I first heard Mike Anderson's, "Healing Cancer from the inside out,"[3] PBS documentary, association of diet with restoring health, I thought, "This is way too good to be true!" I bought two of his books and 2 DVD's, and I read them over and over and over. I looked up the supporting research quoted and concluded that he defended the statements accurately. Anderson often cited T. Colin Campbell's book, *The China Study*. [4] After reading studiously Campbell's book, I concluded, "That's it! We should avoid eating anything from processed or animal-source foods." I have not found a single academic argument against the premise that Phytonutrition (dietary whole plant-foods) is the human adjunct for optimal health, or formally stated, *"Phytonutrition: Finding Fitness For Life."*

---

[3] "Healing Cancer from the inside out," DVD & Book, Mike Anderson
http://www.ravediet.com/
[4] T. Colin Campbell, Thomas M. Campbell, The China Study, Benbella Books, Dallas, Texas (2006).

I tested the Campbell hypothesis by eating only whole plant foods for 30-days. During the first 2-weeks, this dietary experiment was difficult, for I had a strong craving for processed sweets and fats. After 3-weeks, the pangs for no-no's dissipated and I began to experience a new appreciation for rainbow-colored vegetables and fruits. To my surprise, I found that the plant food lifestyle was quite do-able with new tastes for healthy whole plant foods. My energy levels noticeably increased. I noticed sleep state increased in length and depth (8-10 hours). This was a huge difference between the 7-hours previous to the plant food diet. I have always had modestly high cholesterol, 217-232 mg/dL. It is embarrassing to be a practicing board-certified Holistic Nutritionist and have a cholesterol level associated with poor dietary control. This was in spite of numerous attempts to lower cholesterol by dietary modifications. I tried every diet, dietary supplements, and meal plans known to reduce cholesterol under >200 mg/dL, but I never succeeded…After only 30-days on the whole plant food protocol, my cholesterol levels dropped to an all time low, 171 mg/dL. And after 90-days, my total cholesterol plummeted to 151 mg/dL. The fact that this happened to me might be important to you. Why? Cholesterol plays a progressive role in deaths associated with heart disease, cancer, and Alzheimer's' disease. Diet-associated elevated cholesterol is marker for of how foods either enhance health or provoke disease. There is no reason why others cannot also attain the benefits I gained, except that their appetite cravings might compromise compliance. The proof is in the putting…the next step belongs to you.

TABLE OF CONTENTS

CHAPTER I – APPETITE
[AVENUE TO DEATH OR HIGHWAY TO HEALTH?]

The desire to eat starts in the hypothalamus region of the brain. It is stimulated through the vagal-nerve by stress, tension, emotions, or thyroid hormones, which increase metabolism. Eating carbohydrates stimulates hypothalamus-release of a peptide-messenger called "Neuropeptide Y." The release of Neuropeptide Y sends more signals to the appetite center to crave more carbohydrates. This vicious circle is turned on higher and higher by excitement, emotion, or stress, resulting in overeating. When we eat too much, satiety is harder to attain and set higher with each instance. Animal studies confirm of that it is this excess release of Neuropeptide Y that causes obesity. The hypothalamus also senses other hormone-like messengers such as leptin, ghrelin, PYY 3-36, orexin, and cholecystokinin, which may modify the hypothalamic response. They are produced by the digestive tract and adipose tissue. When people are ill, mediator messengers such as tumor necrosis factor-alpha, interleukin-1, & interleukin -6, or corticotropin-releasing hormone reduce appetite cravings. The hypothalamus is considered the area where control of food intake occurs. This view derived from classic experiments in which food intake was studied in rats with lesions in various areas of the brain.

Such studies clearly identified two regions in the hypothalamus that dramatically influence feeding behavior. Both hypothalamic centers are clearly very important in controlling hunger and satiety.[5]

[hunger center). animals with lesions in this area become anorectic and lose weight

[5] By permission, courtesy of Professor R. A. Bowen, Department of Biomedical Sciences, Colorado State University, Biomedical Hypertext, Colorado State University. http://www.vivo.colostate.edu/hbooks/index.html

Ventromedial hypothalamus (*satiety center*): animals with lesions in this area overeat and become obese.

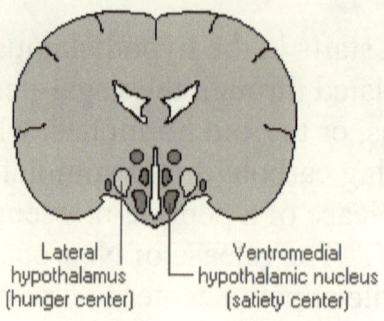

Lateral hypothalamus (hunger center)

Ventromedial hypothalamic nucleus (satiety center)

WHY DO SOME FOODS PROVOKE OVEREATING?
Thoughts of, tastes of, or smells of food stimulate appetite effecting quantity and choices of foods consumed. During eating, the body produces chemosensory signals prior to digestion by triggering salivary, gastric, pancreatic, and intestinal secretions before the food consumed reaches the gut.

Food cravings discriminate what foods are nutritional for meeting a specific transient physiological need. Appetite cravings either resolve a micronutrient deficiency (vitamin or mineral) or they can contribute to calorie-induced obesity. The organ of taste from taste buds is located in the tongue and roof of mouth. Saliva with our sense of smell enables taste perception. Taste is 80-90% of what we smell. To test this, hold your nose, close your eyes, and try to tell the difference between a sliced apple and onion. Each taste bud has a pore that opens out to the surface of the tongue enabling a saliva solution of molecules or ions from foods delivered to receptor cells. All 10,000 taste buds in humans contain between 50-150 receptor cells. A receptor cell lives for 7-14 days, and then, is replaced by a new cell. Each receptor cell in taste buds detects salt, sour, sweet, bitter, umami (or savory fat) tastes. Salt and sour detect taste by <u>ions</u> (from cations and anions), while sweets, bitters, and umami tastes come from <u>molecules</u>. An ion is a molecule in which the total number of electrons is not equal to the total number of protons, giving it a net positive or negative electrical charge. Ions (cations or anions) have a positive or negative charge (+1 or -1), but molecules are neutral.

Thresholds for Taste-Detection are described as follows:

Thresholds Taste-Detection [6]		
Taste	Substance	Substance Threshold
Sweet MOLECULES	Sucrose	0.01 M
Salt IONS	NaCl	0.01 M
Sour IONS	HCL	0.0009 M

---

[6] R. Bowen, Veterinarian Medical School, Colorado State University @:
http://www.vivo.colostate.edu/hbooks/pathphys/digestion/pregastric/taste.html

Umami MOLECULES	Glutamate	0.0007 M
Bitter MOLECULES	Quinine	0.000009 M

Taste preference in the face of specific deficiencies is important. Some examples are removal of the adrenal glands without replacement of mineralocorticoids leads rapidly to death due to massive loss of sodium from the body. Adrenalectomized animals show a clear preference for salt-water over pure water, and if provided with salt water, can actually survive. *Salty taste* drives diet to monitor electrolyte balance. If the parathyroid glands are removed, animals lose calcium and cannot maintain blood calcium levels appropriately due to deficiency in parathyroid hormone.

Following parathyroidectomy, animals choose drinking water that contains calcium chloride over pure water or water containing equivalent concentrations of sodium chloride and avoid salty tastes.

Injection of excess insulin results in hypoglycemia (low blood sugar). Following such, subjects choose the sweetest among foods.

Sweet therefore indicates need for energy nutrients.

Sour is a taste for acids that may occur from alkaline excess, or a warning to avoid a substance due to harmful consequences from a bacteria-spoiled food that has a sour tastes (acidic).

Umami is a craving for amino acids protein needs (e.g. meat, broth, or aged cheese).

Bitter is warning sign to avoid a very bitter taste of diverse harmful natural toxic poison. This is why some dietary supplements or medicines are put in capsules, in order to swallow whole without tasting.

Women are more likely to have specific cravings than men. Women's #1 craving is for chocolate.

Neither men nor women crave low sparse-calorie plant foods. The higher the calorie-density the foods the more it is craved by both men and women.

Hunger increases relative to starvation time.

Hunger increases relative to caloric-depleting exercise. Humans crave salt because we need sodium & chloride from diet.

Men more than women crave amino acid-building blocks for "umami," described as a meaty, savory taste. Dr. Tim Jacobs wrote, "Eating bacon really arouses taste umami receptors because it is a rich source of amino acids."[7] Fat addiction is driven by a complex set of motives to seek pleasure, and avoid pain each of which is associated with survival. The higher the calories per unit of food, the more likely our taste attracts us to eat that food. Rodent studies show they are spontaneously attracted to fat-rich foods.[8] The fat gram contains over double the calories per gram of either carbohydrates or proteins.

Both men and women crave food highest in fat-calories. Johnson & Kenny (2010) show that fat calorie preference is similar to addictive behavior of a cocaine or heroin addict. When they fed rats high-fat junk food, they soon become addicted to the food and voluntarily starved even when given healthy low-fat foods. The fat rats exhibited a self-destructive behavior just like human junkies. Once addicted to a substance, a rodent will starve to death in 10-12 days even when access to healthy foods is available.

---

[7] Professor Tim Jacob, Cardiff University, UK, Taste (Gustation), A tutorial on the sense-of-taste. http://www.cf.ac.uk/biosi/staffinfo/jacob/teaching/sensory/taste.html

[8] Laugerette F, Passilly-Degrace P, Patris B, Niot I, Febbraio M, Montmayeur JP, Besnard P. CD36 involvement in orosensory detection of dietary lipids, spontaneous fat preference, and digestive secretions. J Clin Invest. 2005 Nov;115(11):3177-84.

Humans are born wanting sweets with fats, because carbohydrate provides energy and fat is a calorie-rich survival moiety with addictive behavior effects. As our frequency for eating calorie-dense processed foods increases, so do body fat stores increases. The foods preferred most are those that contain excessive fat and sugar. [9] [10] Researchers also support the notion that over-eating junk food triggers an addictive-compulsive eating pattern. This self-propelling pattern is observed in both obese persons and compulsive drug addicts. [11]

This Self Test helps you to rate the top craved foods:

SELF TEST		
MOST CRAVED FOODS	CALORIES FAT %	CALORIES CARBS %
#1 Chocolate Chip Cookie	50%	46%
#2 Macaroni & Cheese	46%	37%
#3 Milk Chocolate Candy	51%	46%
#4 Chocolate Ice Cream	57%	42%
#5 French Fries	44%	50%
#6 Potato Chips	56%	40%

Survival mechanisms form subconscious influence on how many calories and what kind of calories we consume. Given a choice, research shows that taste always picks the highest calorie foods. [12] [13] [14] Calorie density is a determining factor in survival.

This Self Test permits you testing foods preference based on calorie density:

SELF TEST		
FOOD	CALORIES/ POUND	CALORIE % USA DIET

[9] Drewnowski A, Levine AS. Sugar and fat--from genes to culture. J Nutr. 2003 Mar;133(3):829S-830S.

FATS OILS	4000	93% CALORIES
ICE CREAM	3000	FAVORITES
CHOCOLATE	2500	HIGHLY
POTATO CHIPS	2500	PREFERRED
FRENCH FRIES	2500	
NUTS-SEEDS	2000-2800	
AMERICAN AVERAGE FOOD CHOICE	1500-2000	
CHEESES	1700	
RICE/POTATOES/BEANS	500	7% CALORIES
FRUIT	300	LEAST FAVORITES
VEGETABLES	200	
LEAFY GREENS	100	

Taste is also influenced by how many taste buds we have. Some have a higher number of taste papillae (more taste buds). "Supertasters" have 165 cm^2 taste buds, (25% of the population, more women than men).

Supertasters are less likely to consume the following foods: Brussels sprouts, Cabbage, Kale, Spinach, Soy, Coffee, Grapefruit juice, Green tea, Chili peppers [capsaicin burn is more intense in supertasters], Tonic water [quinine is more bitter to supertasters], Salty olives [for a given concentration, salt is more intense in supertasters], and Alcoholic beverages or Carbonated drinks.

[10] The Facts About Food Cravings by Elaine Magee, MPH, RD, WebMD Weight Loss Clinic - Expert Column @:
http://www.medicinenet.com/script/main/art.asp?articlekey=55942
[11] Johnson PM, Kenny PJ. Dopamine D2 receptors in addiction-like reward dysfunction and compulsive eating in obese rats. Nat Neurosci. 2010 May;13(5):635-41.
[12] Arbour KJ, Wilkie DM. Rodents' (Rattus, Mesocricetus, and Meriones) use of learned caloric information in diet selection. J Comp Psychol. 1988 Jun;102; (2):177-81.
[13] Bolles RC, Hayward L, Crandall C. Conditioned taste preferences based on caloric density. J Exp Psychol Anim Behav Process. 1981 Jan;7(1):59-69.
[14] Warwick ZS, Schiffman SS. Flavor-calorie relationships: effect on weight gain in rats. Physiol Behav. 1991 Sep;50(3):465-70.

"Normal tasters" make up 50% of the population (with 127 cm^2 taste buds), while people with "Poor-to-No taste" sensation (117 cm^2 taste buds) make up the remaining 25% of the population:

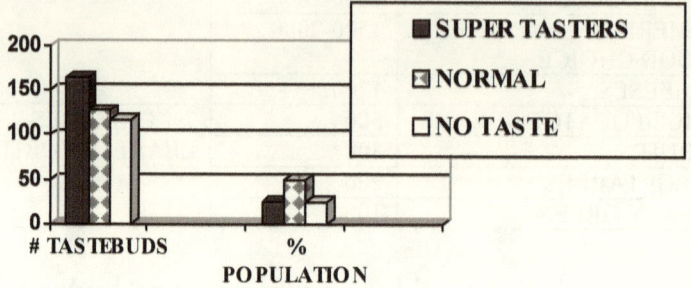

"Normal" and "Super" Tasters are driven toward survival to get enough calories, but because they have more taste buds than "No" tasters, once they taste fat, sweets, and umami flavors, they are challenged to satisfy each taste through pleasure centers by increasing more of each food. Unfortunately, all of the satisfying flavors are inherently calorie-dense resulting in excess fat weight gain. Withdrawal time can take over 1-year, depending on how motivated or how addicted the individual may be:

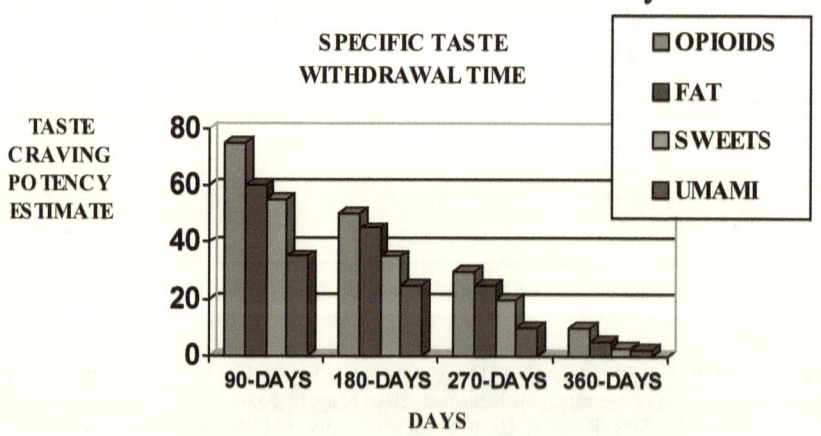

PRACTICAL APPLICATIONS FOR APPETITE CONTROL - What do I do?

People in rural China do not suffer from heart disease or cancers or diabetes like persons in America or developing nations. But if a rural Chinese person moves to or is raised in a developing country, from consuming the same foods as their adopted country, they increase the risk of contracting the same diseases of that nation. You can create a "Country" wherein only healthy foods are permitted. *If a calorie dense fat or sweet food is brought into your home, human behavior pattern demands that it be consumed. If a food is banned from being brought into the home, it will not be eaten.* The following controls* should be adopted for 90-days in order to suppress appetite-induced over-eating by establishing separation from the problem, i.e. isolation to "Country" wherein a healthy nutrition lifestyle is law: [15]

*Remove any food, drink, or herb that stimulates appetite. Specific examples are alcoholic drinks, fruit juices, processed foods, refined sugars, high fat foods, meats, dairy products, Aniseed, Artichoke leaf, Barberry, Bitter melon, Blessed thistle, Cardamom seeds, Catnip, Chamomile, Daikon, Fennel Fenugreek seeds, Gentian, Juniper (berries), Parsley, Spearmint, and Watercress.

*Sleep is a required appetite suppressant; adequate sleep induces appetite control. People who do not sleep well increase the hormone, ghrelin, which is shown to increase appetite.

---

[15] This protocol should followed with strict compliance for 90-days.

*Hydration of 8-10 fluid ounces water 30 minutes before each meal will suppress appetite. Water is a safe appetite-suppressant that supports optimal metabolic rate. Hydration enables kidneys to flush out the toxins and other waste materials from the body. Dehydration increases appetite and turns off fat metabolism.

*Fiber should be the first food eaten during a meal to absorb water and expand in stomach. Foods high in fiber require more energy for digestion. Eating a salad first before your meal with herbs will suppress appetite. Salads consisting of cabbage, spinach and endives are appetite suppressors.

*Soup suppresses appetite for weight loss and appetite control; they are low in calories and have high water content.

*Apples are natural appetite suppressants with anti-inflammatory properties that reportedly reduce cravings. A fiber-rich apple requires more time to chew and digest causing a full feeling.

*Flaxseeds (ground) are an effective appetite suppressant, high-fiber and rich in omega-3 fatty acids. An ounce of flaxseeds provides 8-grams fiber that inhibits rise in blood sugar and reduces several hormones from stimulating hunger pangs.

*Oatmeal is a healthy, high-fiber, low-glycemic carbohydrate for breakfast that results in appetite-control for hours.

*Addiction to high-fat or processed sweet calories can require 90-days abstinence to resolve. Avoid all fatty foods, processed foods, or foods containing MSG or umami-flavoring additives.

CONCLUSION: Appetite, cravings, including our individual taste preferences is tightly controlled by habit. It is proven that when a person on a calorie-sparse whole plant food diet moves to an area where calorie-dense processed, high-fat, high-processed sugars are consumed, they adopt not only the diet but also the diseases common to that area. Appetite can be retrained within 30 to 90-days. Benefits are soon confirmed by body fat weight loss, increased energy level, enhanced mental acuity, and decreased total cholesterol.

CHAPTER II - THE CHINA STUDY – Nutrient Associations Health & Disease

The China Study, conducted by T. Colin Campbell and his colleagues, is the most comprehensive study of nutrition ever. This enormous research studied nutrient associations with health and disease in 6,500 people in 130 villages across China between the ages 35-64. They looked at a wide variety of 367 variables from three-day dietary intake questionnaire was used to collect information about Chinese dietary lifestyle. Blood and urine samples were also collected and analyzed to eliminate bias from the subjective dietary intake questionnaire. Nutrients were compared by the amount consumed, blood born substances, and metabolites excreted in the urine.

The Dietary Lifestyles differences between Americans and Chinese:

America compared to China		
AREA	AMERICA	CHINA
Calorie average per day	1989	2641
Body Mass Index average	27.0	21.0
Total Fat (% of calories)	36%	14.5%
Dietary Fiber (grams/day)	12	33
Total Protein (grams/day)	91	64
AREA	AMERICA	CHINA
Protein Sources	70% Animal 30% Vegetable (Protein is 11.0% of all calories)	10% Animal 90% Vegetable (Protein is 0.8 % of all calories)
Total Iron (mg/day)	18	34
Cholesterol Ranges	170-290 mg/dL	90-170 mg/dL
Total Cholesterol Averages	199 mg/dL	127 mg/dL
Menarche-Menopause Age Range	12-51.0	15-48
Lifetime Estrogen Exposure Estimate %	100%	50%

The China Study reported nutrient associations with health and disease*:
*Calorie intake is 30% higher in rural China as compared to the United States.

*Chinese Body average Mass Index is a healthy 21.0, yet they consume 652 calories more per day than Americans.
*Americans have an obese 27.0 Body Mass Index, in spite of eating -652 less calories less per day than Chinese.
*Cancers have been associated with higher dietary fat intake.
*Americans consume 1/3rd of the dietary fiber of the Chinese.
*Fiber intake is 3-times higher in China than in the USA and it correlates with a lower rate of colon and rectal cancers in China.
Diseases of affluence, Coronary Heart Disease, Diabetes, Colon Cancer, Lung Cancer, Leukemia, Childhood Brain Cancer, Stomach Cancer, and Liver Cancer tend to increase as the cholesterol levels increase.
*Americans diet of animal foods increase ⬆ cholesterol, while plant foods of Chinese result in a decrease in ⬇ cholesterol.
*Heart disease is not observed in Chinese with total cholesterol levels of less than 150 mg/dL. Do our Genes or Lifestyle cause disease?
*When rural Chinese move to America, their genes do not change, but due to adopted changes in dietary-lifestyle, they take on the same disease pattern of Americans.
*The China Study concludes that a whole plant food diet reduces disease-state and improves health compared to consuming an animal-sourced (red meat and white meat, dairy, fish) foods diet in America.

The following table lists the major effects from and differences between Americans, who eat mostly animal-source foods compared to the Chinese, who eat mostly plant source foods:

CHARACTERISTICS ANIMAL VERSUS PLANT FOODS [16]		
CHARACTERISTIC	ANIMAL-FOODS[17]	PLANT-FOODS[18]
Effect of protein-type to catalyze cholesterol-induced atherosclerosis	Yes Trend to increase ↑	No Trend to decrease ↓
Effect on total blood cholesterol	Trend to increase ↑ (170-290 mg/dL in Western society)	Trend to decrease ↓ (90-150 mg/dL in China)
Effect on Body Mass Index (BMI)	High BMI	Low BMI
Saturated fat	Yes	No
Polyunsaturated fats & Unsaturated fats	No	Yes
High structural volume complex carbohydrate	No	Yes
High structural content protein & fat	Yes	No
Lifetime estrogen exposure	Trend to increase ↑ estrogen lifetime exposure 200% (Onset-early menarche & delayed menopause)	Trend to decrease ↓ estrogen lifetime exposure 50% of animal-sourced foods (Delayed menarche & early menopause)
Effect of calories on body fat storage	Trend to increase ↑	Trend to decrease ↓
Effect of calories on metabolism	Trend to decrease ↓	Trend to increase ↑
Effect of whole foods on disease	As animal protein increases (above 12% k/cal), cholesterol levels and onset of disease increases ↑	As plant food increases cholesterol levels and onset of disease decreases ↓
Antioxidants	None	Yes
Fiber grams per 500 k/cal	None	31 grams
Cholesterol per 500 k/cal	137 mg	None
Fat gram per 500 k/cal	36 grams	4 grams
Betacarotene mcg per 500 k/cal	0.017 mg	29.9 mg
Vitamin C mg per 500 k/cal	4 mg	293 mg
Folate mg per 500 k/cal	0.019 mg	1.16 mg
Vitamin E mg/ATE per 500 k/cal	0.5 mg/ATE	11 mg/ATE
Iron mg per 500 k/cal	20 mg	0.5 mg

[16] Campbell TC. Campbell TM. *The China Study*. Benbella Books. Dallas, Texas.
[17] Equal parts of beef, pork, chicken, & whole milk.
[18] Equal parts of tomatoes, spinach, lima beans, peas, & potatoes.

Magnesium mg per 500 k/cal	61 mg	548 mg
Calcium mg per 500 k/cal	252 mg	545 mg

When animal source calories dominate menu, the harmful effects are increases in obesity, BMI, total cholesterol, and estrogen, which may compromise health. It is that simple.

CALORIE ASSOCIATIONS WITH HEALTH & MORTALITY

Eating too many calories is associated with obesity. Statistics show weight, and lifestyle trends from 1970-2007, indicate that obesity doubled in the USA. [19]

Americans eating fewer calories than rural Chinese but more than they need increases the rate of obesity and risk of compromised health.

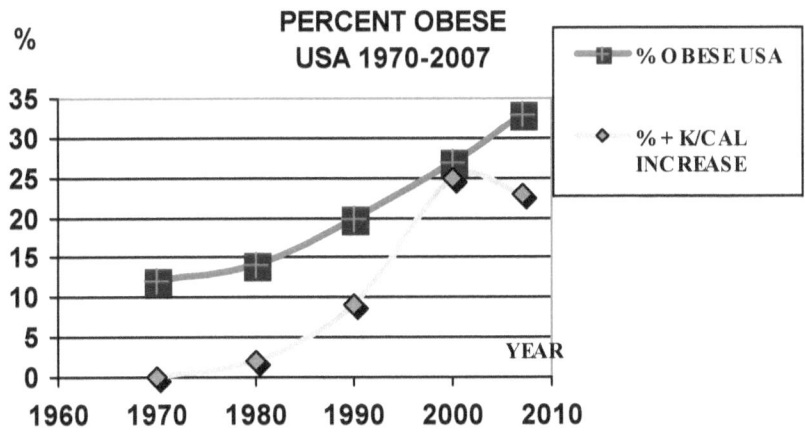

PERCENT OBESE USA 1970-2007

[19] Extrapolated from charts posted by Dr. Stephan Guyenet Ph.D., Whole Health Source. Data from the National Health and Nutrition Examination Survey (NHANES), the Behavioral Risk Factor Surveillance System (BRFSS), and the U.S. Department of Agriculture (USDA).
http://wholehealthsource.blogspot.com/2008/12/us-weight-lifestyle-and-diet-trends.html

In the USA, increases in calories originated from meats, fats, and refined sugars, not from whole plant foods. Notice below, that the rate of obesity closely parallels meats and fat consumption.

Surprisingly, the -2% decrease in total calories (the only decrease) between 2000-2007 did not reduce the rate of obesity; it increased obesity from 27% to 33%.

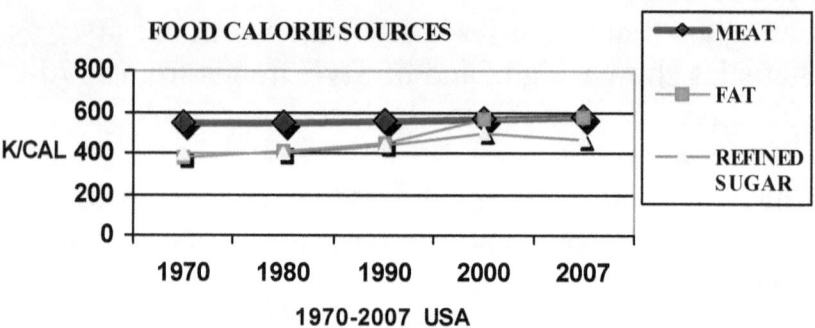

This information implies that obesity's onset and potential threat to health issues could be preventable at mealtime…. Obesity has been identified as the #2 preventable cause of death (below), sandwiched between cigarette smoking and alcohol.

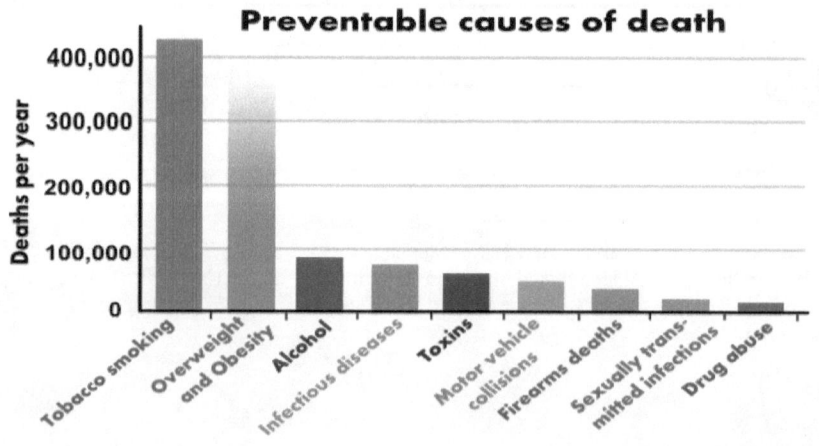

Obesity (by comparison) contributes to more premature deaths than all the infectious diseases, toxins, motor vehicle deaths, firearm deaths, sexually transmitted deaths, and drug abuse combined. [20]

A Healthy body mass index ranges between 18.5-25.0. The average American today has an obese body mass index of 27.0 and shows no sign of decreasing to a healthy normal BMI; see table on page 19. [21]

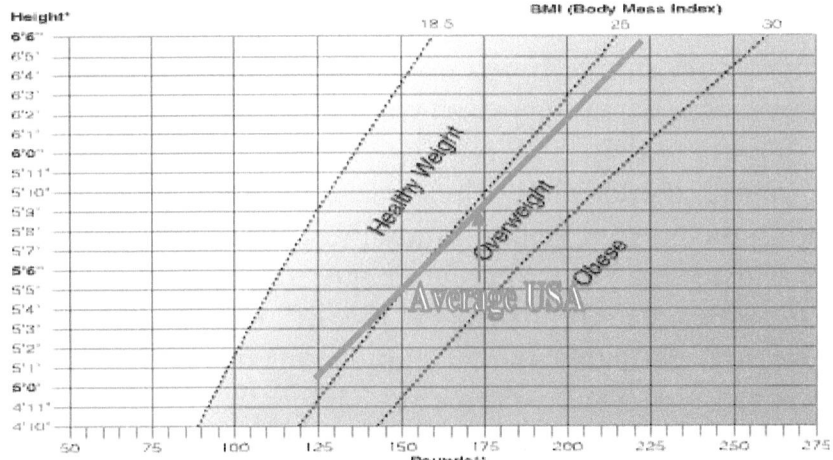

PRACTICAL APPLICATIONS FROM THE CHINA STUDY - What do I do?[*]

The whole plant food dietary lifestyle (as studied in rural China) is associated with a reduced onset of diseases associated with intake animal food dietary lifestyle (in America).

[20] Mokdad AH, Marks JS, Stroup DF, Gerberding JL (March 2004). "Actual causes of death in the United States, 2000". *JAMA* **291** (10): 1238–45.
[21] Source: National Institutes of Health

*The goal of a healthy diet is total cholesterol under 150 mg/dL, low body mass index BMI<25.0, and energy levels to include 30-60 minutes exercise daily.

*Chinese consume 652 more calories average daily than Americans; their slim BMI of 21.0 is only 3/4th of obese Americans' 27.0 BMI. This concludes that plant food calories increase energy, basal metabolism rate, and burn more efficiently than animal-source calories.

*Americans consume an average range of 35-40% of their total calories from fat.

*Chinese consume an average range of 14.5% of their total calories from fat.

*There is a 90% correlation between total fat and animal protein intake; fat intake increases parallel with animal protein from animal-based foods.

*Breast cancer rate increases with total intake of animal fat, but not with plant-fats.

*A low-fat diet does not always lead to lower breast cancer risk. In the Nurses' Health Study there was no evidence that a lower intake of total fat or specific major types of fat were associated with decreased risk of breast cancer. The decrease in fat intake in this study showed and associated increase in animal food proteins. This indicates an association with the proportion of animal-based foods consumed by those who have a higher risk of cancer.

*A whole-food plant-based diet reduces the risk of diabetes, breast cancer, colon cancer, and cardiovascular diseases, and stroke.

Recommendation: Remove all animal-based calories and refined sugars from the diet for 90-days to initiate new dietary lifestyle. Why 90-days? Based on reports from the Monell Chemical Senses Center, 90-days fasting fats, sugars, and meats is required to eliminate cravings. Once completed, taste and cravings change toward eating a variety of whole plant-foods.

CHAPTER III FATS
Nutrient Associations with Health or Disease

What are the effects associated with NOT eating animal fats? Persons living in rural China (from The China Study), Papua Highlands in New Guinea, those living in central Africa, or Tarahumara Indians living in northern Mexico do not eat high-calorie processed fatty rich foods. They are perfectly content to eat a whole plant food menu! Interestingly they do not suffer from cardiovascular disease (or cancers). Bring any one of them in to our culture and let them sample the American menu, and they take on our disease patterns in time. Conversely, when a total whole plant food diet is introduced and animal foods are restricted from a population, the death rate from cardiovascular diseases is dramatically reduced. In 1940-1945, World War II, the Germans confiscated all Norway's cattle, sheep, goats, pigs, chickens and chickens to feed the soldiers. The Norwegians were forced to exist on only whole plant-based foods. This graphic picture on the following page shows the remarkable decrease in Norway's death rates from heart disease when they were forced to consume a whole plant food menu...

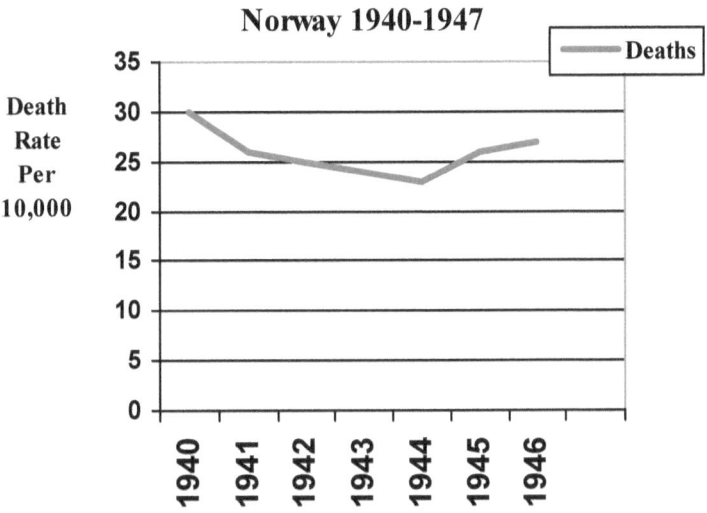

Deaths Cardiovascular Heart Disease Norway 1940-1947

Death Rate Per 10,000

Notice that after only 1-year on a whole plant food diet that 4000 less people died from cardiovascular heart disease or stroke in Norway. After 4 years time had passed, 7000 less Norwegians were dying from circulatory disease each year. Though the Germans did not mean to save Norwegians by taking away their animal sourced foods, 31,000 fewer Norwegians died from circulatory diseases during 1940-1945 than died previously from 1935-1940 when they consumed animal foods. [22]

FATTY FOODS FORM PLAQUES IN ARTERIES HEART DISEASE

Plaque formation starts in the lining of the artery shown as a tear, trauma, or insult.

[22] TCC502 Dr. Esselstyn Lecture notes from eCornell Plant Food Certificate Course @:http://www.ecornell.com/certificate-programs/personal-interest-training/certificate-in-plant-based-nutrition-certificate/crt/TCCC01

The body can make its own cholesterol to meet its own soft tissue and hormonal needs; therefore a dietary source is not required. Once Cholesterol levels in the blood are higher than required, the rate of plaque **formation on artery walls** may result in plaque buildup that could contribute to heart disease, (atherosclerosis).

Excess blood cholesterol commonly occurs from eating animal foods (meats, eggs, poultry, fish, and dairy products). Blood cholesterol is closely associated with the amount of total animal food fat or saturated fat in the diet; saturated fat raises blood cholesterol proportionate to diet dose. Whole plant foods do not contain cholesterol.

Progression of plaque build-up in coronary artery

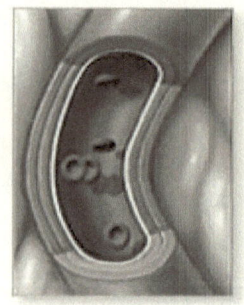

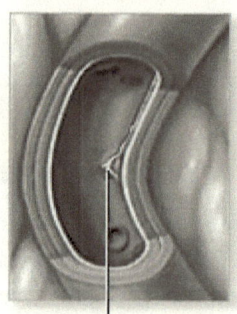

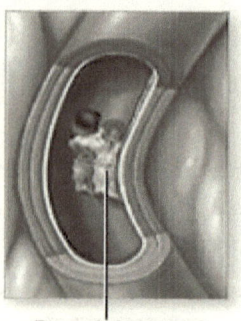

Normal

Tear in lining of artery

Fat and cholesterol accumulate

ADAM.[23] [24]

Normal actual coronary artery progressing toward coronary artery disease (atherosclerosis) shows marked luminal narrowing.

[23] Reviewed By: Steven Kang, MD, Division of Cardiac Pacing and Electrophysiology, Cardiovascular Consultants Medical Group, Oakland, CA. Review provided by VeriMed Healthcare Network. http://healthguide.howstuffworks.com/progressive-build-up-of-plaque-in-coronary-artery-picture.htm

[24] Reviewed By: Steven Kang, MD, Division of Cardiac Pacing and Electrophysiology, Cardiovascular Consultants Medical Group, Oakland, CA. Review provided by VeriMed Healthcare Network. http://healthguide.howstuffworks.com/progressive-build-up-of-plaque-in-coronary-artery-picture.htm

Plaque accumulation deposits over time with elevated cholesterol.[25]

Similar plaque-formation in artery walls compares a normal to a plaque-diseased artery.

BIRTH OF A PLAQUE

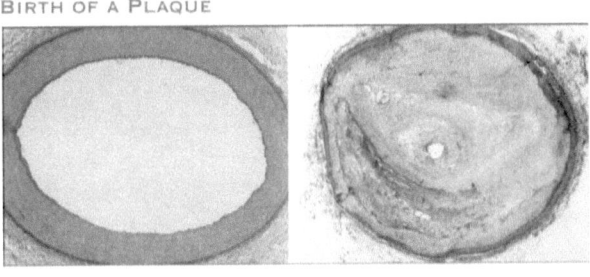

Normal Artery   Diseased Artery

Actual healthy-normal ↑ artery compared to ↑ a diseased artery [26] Coronary artery disease is a condition in which plaque builds up inside the coronary arteries. These arteries supply the heart muscle with oxygen-rich blood. Plaque is made up of fat, cholesterol, calcium, and other substances found in the blood. When plaque builds up in the walls of arteries, a condition is called Atherosclerosis results. (On the next page see Figure A showing a normal artery with normal blood flow. Figure B shows an artery with plaque buildup.) Plaque narrows the arteries and reduces blood flow to the heart.

[25] World Health Organization @ http://apps.who.int/classifications/apps/icd/icd10online/?gi20.htm+i20
[26] TCC502 from Dr. Esselstyn's Lecture, Courtesy of Dr. Caldwell Esselstyn and eCornell Plant Food Certificate Course @: http://www.ecornell.com/certificate-programs/personal-interest-training/certificate-in-plant-based-nutrition-certificate/crt/TCCC01

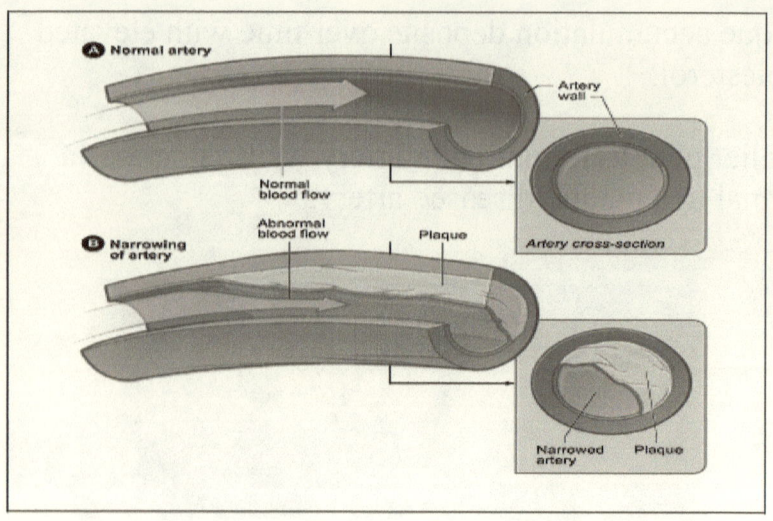

It also makes it more likely that blood clots will form in your arteries. Blood clots can partially or completely block blood flow. [27] Diseased clogged arteries account for only 10% of the heart attacks. While clogging due to plaque narrowing on outer edge of the artery walls is harmful, the most dangerous form causing the remaining 90% is the form of plaque that ruptures free flapping off the artery wall and may free plaques of size into the blood stream. The picture on the next page shows how a plaque-rupture either impedes blood flow or releases plaque material into the bloodstream. [28]

[27] National Institute of Health @:
http://www.nhlbi.nih.gov/health/dci/Diseases/Cad/CAD_All.html
[28] TCC502 Dr. Esselstyn Lecture notes, courtesy of Dr. Caldwell Esselstyn from the eCornell Plant Food Certificate Course @: http://www.ecornell.com/certificate-programs/personal-interest-training/certificate-in-plant-based-nutrition-certificate/crt/TCCC01

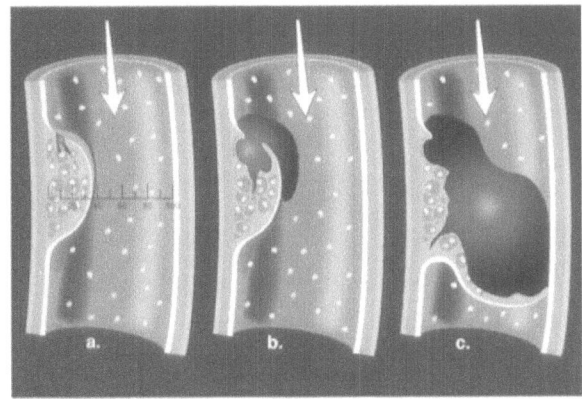

Clogging of the Arteries

The pressure of blood against the walls of blood vessels is enough to free the plaque material to cause a blockage or rupture of plaque material. A heart attack occurs when an area of plaque in a coronary artery breaks apart, causing a blood clot to form. The blood clot cuts off most or all blood to the part of the heart muscle that's fed by that artery. Cells in the heart muscle downstream die because they don't receive enough oxygen-rich blood damaging the heart. [29]

[29] National Institute of Health @:
http://www.nhlbi.nih.gov/health/dci/Diseases/Cad/CAD_All.html

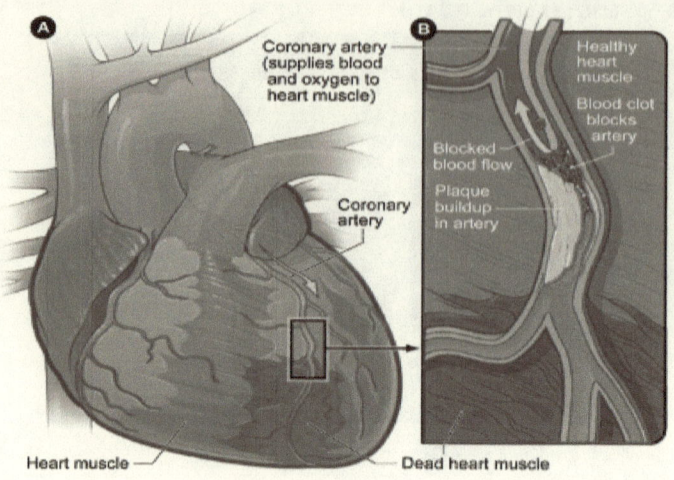

A

Coronary artery
(supplies blood
and oxygen to
heart muscle)

Healthy
heart
muscle

B

Blood clot
blocks
artery

Blocked
blood flow

Coronary
artery

Plaque
buildup
in artery

Heart muscle

Dead heart muscle

DIETARY FAT ASSOCIATED WITH CARDIOVASCULAR HEART DISEASE

There is an association between eating too much fat and serum cholesterol effects associated with cardiovascular heart disease. [30]. Clogging vascular wall surfaces with tiny plaque deposits reduces blood flow volume, inhibits waste removal, restricts nutrient delivery, limits oxygen exchange, and reduces optimal blood flow. In the sedentary population, cardiovascular performance declines progressively with age. However, much of this decline may be attributed to physical inactivity and increased body fat. Maximal oxygen consumption values decline in sedentary subjects at -10% per decade after age 25. However, if body composition is maintained by physical activity and a healthy low-fat diet, the decline in VO^2max due to aging is slowed to 4-5% per decade. This decline can be less; as little as 1-2% per decade, if exercise is performed regularly and a healthy low-fat whole plant food is consumed.

THIN PLAQUE LAYER REDUCES BLOOD FLOW VOLUME

It is mathematically possible that a 2-millimeter thin layer of plaque added to a vascular wall surface will inhibit the rate of blood flow. If a healthy coronary artery 10-mm wide is reduced to 8-mm, this represents huge -56% total blood flow volume loss. Blood Volume Loss in Artery Diameter Artery = 56% Less volume:

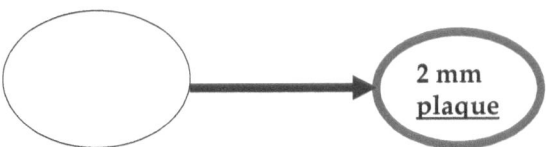

REDUCED BLOOD OXYGEN STIMULATES VASODILATION RESPONSE

Scientists also discovered that when they applied a blood pressure cuff to the upper arm slightly above systolic blood pressure level for 5-minutes, upon releasing the cuff, the arteries in the forearm dilated and refilled. [31] What causes this? Nitric oxide is produced following anoxia, which stimulates "vasoactivity" or vasodilation in blood vessels for an increased blood flow return. Exercise will increase the efficacy of the NO-pathway by physically expanding, contracting, and stretching vascular epithelial walls. Following a warm up before exercise, movement is attained with less effort. EXAMPLE: Start running at race pace for a few minutes, then rest for a minute and repeat at the same pace. Note how much easier it is the second time…this is due to an increase in nitric oxide to relax artery wall diameters! This effects of nitric oxide NO-released from epithelial cells in the lining of blood vessels relax vessels to dilate and expand, increase blood flow volume.

---

[31] Vogel RA, Corretti MC, Plotnick GD. Effect of a single high-fat meal on endothelial

The artery-vasodilator NO acts to increase intracellular release of a substance called EDRF and thus the activation of the cGMP signal cascade. EDRF is the free radical diatomic gas, nitric oxide, NO. NO is formed by the action of NO synthase, (NOS) on the amino acid, Arginine (chart): [32]

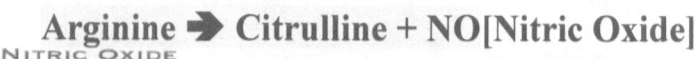

Arginine ➔ Citrulline + NO[Nitric Oxide]

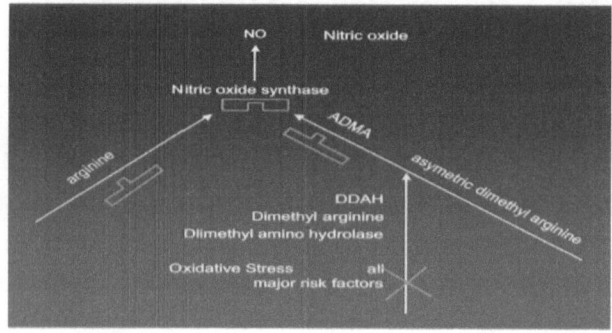

The Nitric Oxide pathway is created by epithelial cells in the lining of arteries in order to relax and open arteries to increase oxygen and glucose to working muscles in need of replenishment and waste removal. Regular exercise improves the efficiency of the Nitric Oxide pathway. However, when blood fats increase, the nitric oxide pathway is turned off. Keeping blood fat low therefore is always recommended. The more efficient the nitric oxide pathway, the better the blood flow volume return.

---

function in healthy subjects. Am J Cardiol. 1997 Feb 1;79(3):350-4.
[32] TCC502 Dr. Esselstyn Lecture notes, courtesy of eCornell Plant Food Certificate Course @: http://www.ecornell.com/certificate-programs/personal-interest-training/certificate-in-plant-based-nutrition-certificate/crt/TCCC01

Vogel[33] also showed that the higher the fasting LDL-cholesterol is before exercise, the lower the NO flow-mediated activity. Having low fasting total cholesterol levels sets a circulatory environment conducive to performance gains. LDL-cholesterol is named "Bad Cholesterol" because, when oxidized, it makes vessel walls "sticky with plaques" thereby increasing progressive risk of atherogenic disease. Scientists measured a single high fat-meal of 50 grams fat and demonstrated that it negatively inhibited NO-vasodilatation on blood flow volume. [34] They utilized a sophisticated ultrasound device to measure the effect of fat or carbohydrate calories on epithelial cell nitric oxide cascade on artery diameter increase. They gave subjects either a NO FAT MEAL consisting of Frosted Flakes breakfast cereal, skim milk, and orange juice or a HIGH FAT (50 grams fat) meal consisting of an Egg Mcmuffin-Sausage meal with hash browns. The next chart shows an inhibitory effect from consuming a high fat meal versus a no-fat meal intake on blood flow volume up to 4-hours after eating. [35]

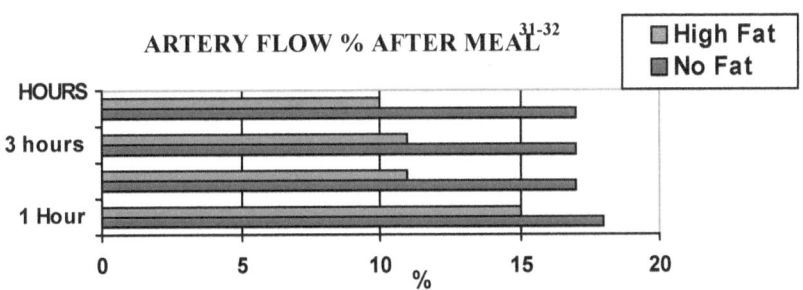

[33] Ibid. Vogel RA, et al., Am J Cardiol. 1997 Feb 1;79(3):350-4.
[34] Vogel RA, Corretti MC, Plotnick GD. Effect of a single high-fat meal on endothelial function in healthy subjects. Am J Cardiol. 1997 Feb 1;79(3):350-4.
[35] Ibid.

While a single meal may not be fatal, the repeated effects from fat on inhibited blood flow may have consequences. Over a 10-year period consumption of an average 55-117 grams of fat per day may raise individual total cholesterol levels significantly. Diet frequency from 11,000 meals 55-117 grams of fat per day could impose a minimum of 605,000 grams to a maximum of 1,287,000 grams of dietary fat. Dietary fats consumed will proportionately increase blood lipids with increased rate of plaque accumulation on blood vessel walls. The following dietary factors increase cholesterol levels coffee, butter, margarine, all fats (extracted oils, meats, dairy), trans-fatty acids, fructose, sucrose, and alcohol.[36] Reducing all high-fat, addictive foods accomplishes an improved circulatory delivery of copious amounts of oxygen, calories, fluids, and electrolytes to supply all living cell tissue sites. Consuming a high-pH, antioxidant-rich, high-fiber whole plant food menu results in cholesterol-reducing benefits. [37] Consuming foods high in fat inhibit the Nitric Oxide cascade and eventually the impact of 10-years meals of 605,000-1,287,000 grams of fat may contribute to plaque accumulation on artery walls. The more plaque, the less blood flows past the deposit sites on artery walls. Optimal blood flow volume is associated with health. Reduced blood flow volume is associated with onset of systemic cardiovascular disease. [38]

---

[36] Besides diet, stress, hypothyroidism, menopause, anabolic-androgenic steroids, and not exercising may also increase cholesterol levels.

[37] The Author reduced his total cholesterol from 232 to 151 mg/DL after 150 days following a 100% plant food diet.

[38] Maton, Anthea (1995). Human Biology Health. Englewood Cliffs, New Jersey: Prentice Hall. ISBN 0-13-981176-1.

ESSELSTYN'S "NO-FAT" CALORIES POSITION

For nutrition to support optimal health, elimination of all high fat foods, all meats, oils, nuts, and seeds is recommended. Dr. Caldwell Esselstyn's nutrition position stance for "NO-FAT" is very well defended. Why no fat? We learned earlier that CD36 receptors in the brain crave fat like an addict craves an opioid drug. Once the CD36 receptor experiences satisfaction once, it then craves more in order return to its former satiated status. When blood lipids from a single meal increase, they turn off the nitric oxide pathway inhibiting circulation flow rate for up to 2.5 hours. Repeating meals that contain more than 18 grams fat will impact blood circulation negatively with each incidence.

Over a 24-hour period our body requires only 11-grams total fat, 2 grams of omega-3 and 9 grams of omega-6 fatty acids to meet the daily essential fat requirement. [39] Omega-3 is an anti-inflammatory fatty acid the body cannot make. Omega-6 is a pro-inflammatory fat the body cannot make, but omega-6 fats are added to breads, spreads, packaged, and processed foods may create excess amounts. When an omega-6 and omega-3 are consumed together, the ideal ratio is 1:1, 2:1, or 3:1. O-6 and O-3 utilize a common enzyme enroute through digestion-metabolic processing. If the two essential fats are consumed at the same time, the fat that is highest will inhibit absorption of the one that is lower. Common oils typically generate an unhealthy Omega 6 to Omega 3 ratio; examples are olive oil is 13:1, sunflower oil is 15:1, and corn oil is 79:1.

---

[39] American Heart Association's recommended upper limit is 8% saturated fat calories based on a 2000 calorie/day diet means a total of 160 calories or 18 grams saturated fat per day.

Even the essential fatty O6:O3-ratios of nuts and seeds is unhealthy ranging from 4:1 to 1800:1. When dietary fat ratio favors Omega-6 above the 3:1, an increased risk of blood clots, artery constriction, inflammatory arthritis, IGF-1-hormone (cancer risk), excess insulin, excess blood sugar, obesity, and psoriasis skin irritation may result. Most American diets average between 20:1 and 30:1 Omega-6 to Omega-3 fat. There are two foods that provide a healthy fat Omega-6:Omega-3 ratio, Flaxseeds 1:3.6 and Macadamia Nuts 1:1.

ESSELSTYN'S REMARKABLE RESULTS [40]

When Dr. Esselstyn finished with a 4-hour counseling session with a triple-bypass heart patient, they were well convinced to employ drastic changes in both their diet and lifestyle. Here is a graphic presentation of their results after employing his "NO-FAT" position to their diet. It took approximately 90-days for each person to overcome their desire to eat fat foods.

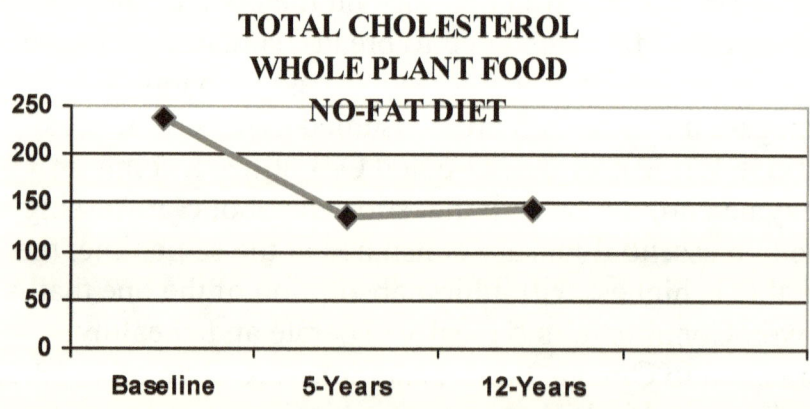

TOTAL CHOLESTEROL
WHOLE PLANT FOOD
NO-FAT DIET

WHOLE PLANT FOOD DIET

[40] TCC502 Dr. Esselstyn Lecture notes, courtesy of eCornell Plant Food Certificate Course @: http://www.ecornell.com/certificate-programs/personal-interest-training/certificate-in-plant-based-nutrition-certificate/crt/TCCC01

REVERSES BLOCKED ARTERIES

Even more convincing and impressive is what happened inside heart patient's blocked arteries (below) after they went on a "NO-FAT" whole plant food diet:

➢ A 67-year old Pediatrician 1987-1992.
➢ A 58-year old Factory Worker 1985-1992.
➢ A 54-year old Security Guard 1987-1992.
➢ A 44-year old Surgeon 1996-1999.

(1) A 67-year old Pediatrician 1987-1992.

REVERSAL OF CORONARY DISEASE

1987   1992

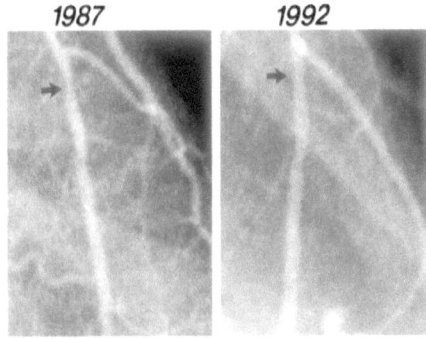

Coronary Angiograms

(2) A 58-year old Factory Worker 1985-1992.

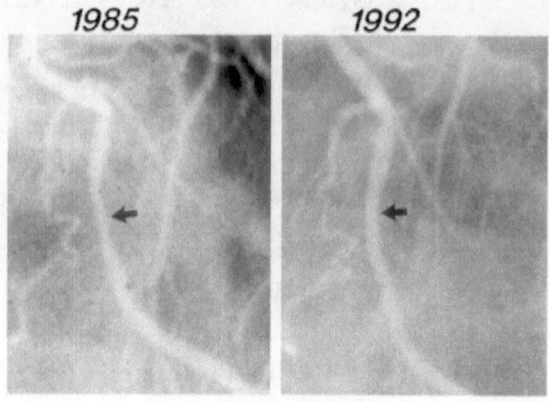

Factory Worker
58 Years Old

(3) A 54-year old Security Guard 1987-1992.

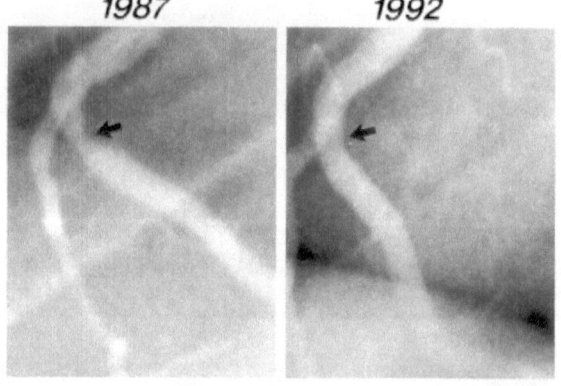

Security Guard
54 Years Old

(4) A 44-year old Surgeon 1996-1999.

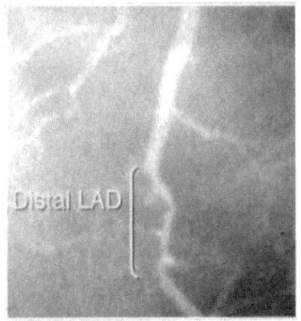 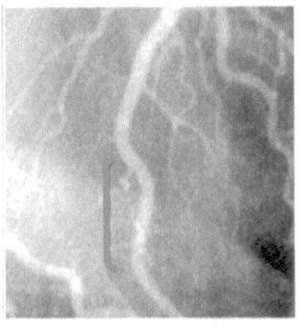

November 27, 1996   July 22, 1999

Esselstyn also showed PET Scans of cross sections of 4 patients' hearts of before and after only 14-days on a whole plant food diet with "No Fats."

Each of 4-subjects improved circulatory flow patterns are pictured as bright red through the heart muscle:
>1. 58-year old School Bus Driver Cholesterol dropped -135 points.
>2. 75-year old Retired Tool & Die Maker Cholesterol dropped -111 points.
>3. 65-year old Barber Cholesterol dropped -160 points.
>4. 58-year old Stock Broker Cholesterol dropped -111 points.

(1) 58-year old School Bus Driver.

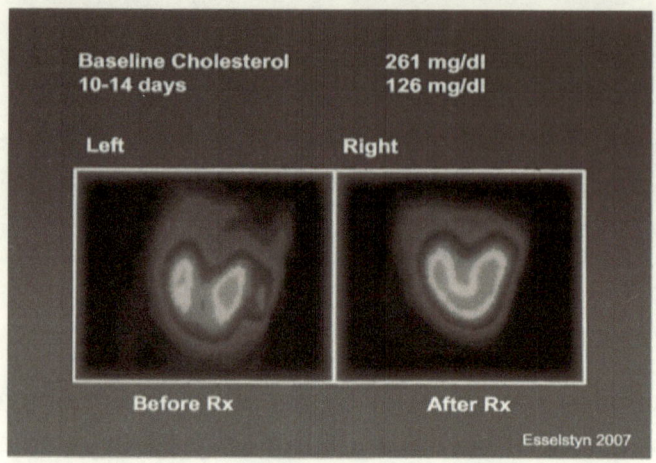

(2) 75-year old Retired Tool & Die Maker.

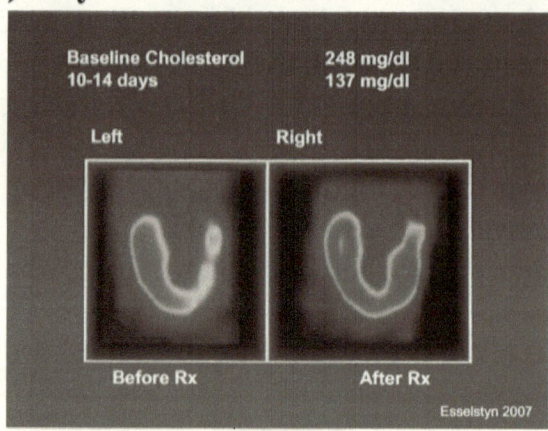

Retired Tool Maker

(3) 65-year old Barber.

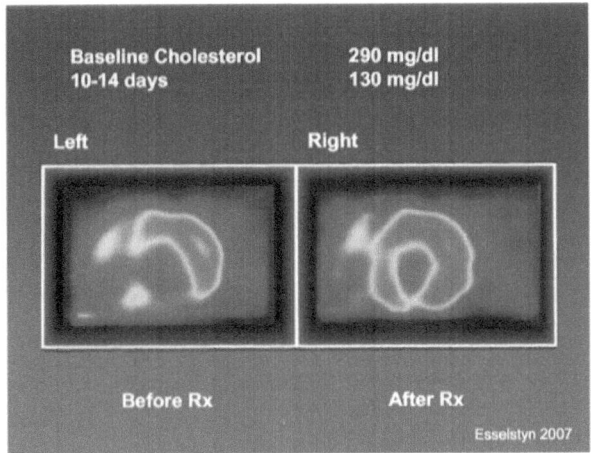

Retired Barber
65 Years Old

(4) 58-year old Stock Broker.

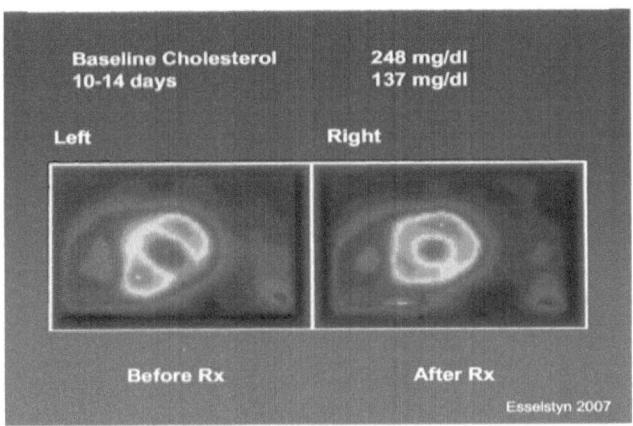

Stock Broker
58 Years Old

PLANT FOOD DIET EFFECTS ARE MEASURED IN DAYS

While it may take 90-days to overcome the craving for fats, when compliance is strictly followed, it only takes 14-21 days for remarkable effects to occur. The four subjects (above) each lowered their total cholesterol levels from 111-160 points in 14 days. Others reported positive healthy changes in (1) Diabetic Blood Sugar levels and (2) Osteoporosis, Blood Calcium levels in only a few days [see diagram]: [41] [42] [43]

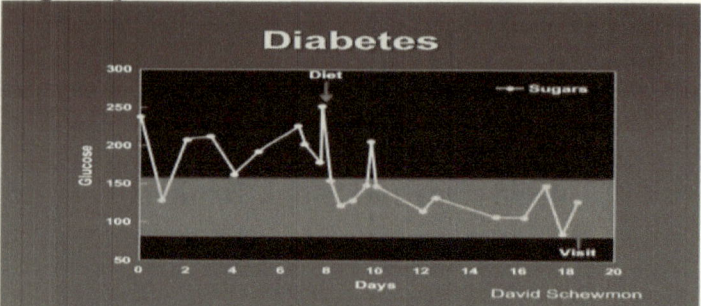

Diabetic Patient Back to Normal After Plant Based Diet

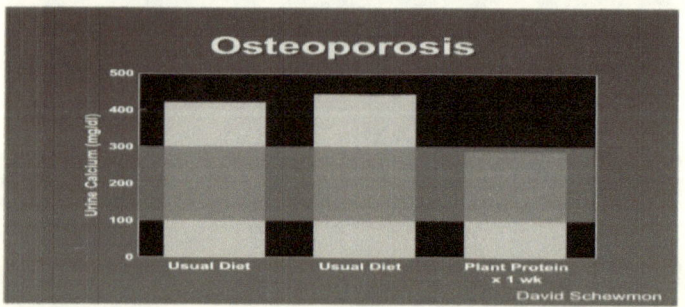

Urinary Calcium Back to Normal After Plant Based Diet

---

[41] Diabetes & Osteoporosis Blood Sugar and Blood Calcium changes after Plant Food diet by permission courtesy of T. Colin Campbell Foundation, from TCC502 Lecture on Autoimmune diseases @ http://www.ecornell.com/certificate-programs/personal-interest-training/certificate-in-plant-based-nutrition-certificate/crt/TCCC02
[42] Lecture TCC502 eCornell Plant Food Certificate Course, By permission, courtesy of Dr. T. Colin Campbell @: http://www.tcolincampbell.org/
[43] Ibid. By permission, courtesy of Dr. T. Colin Campbell: http://www.tcolincampbell.org/

PRACTICAL APPLICATIONS FOR ANIMAL VERSUS PLANT – What do I do?

➤ A whole plant food diet without added or excess fat calories [44] lowers total cholesterol in 10-14 days.

➤ A whole plant food diet without added or excess fat calories improves heart blood flow volume in 10-14 days.

➤ A whole plant food diet without added or excess fat calories improves blood sugar levels within 3-8 days.

➤ A whole plant food diet without added or excess fat calories improves blood calcium levels within 7 days.

➤ A whole plant food diet without added or excess fat calories improves blood circulation immediately after a meal.

➤ A whole plant food diet without added or excess fat calories may require 90-days application to reduce learned fat-calorie cravings.

➤ Bring only whole plant foods into the home. What foods are allowed in the home are the foods that will be consumed. If only plant foods are brought into the living quarters for 90-days, then only plant foods will be consumed.

➤ Expect actual results in 10-14 days, but do not expect lifestyle cravings to change appreciably until after 90-days fasting craved foods. It takes time to change a habit, but it can be done.

---

[44] "No fat" amount of dietary is not well defined since no research has examined beyond dietary effect less than 50-grams fat on Vogel's brachial artery test for nitric oxide vasodilatation response. Nevertheless, Esselstyn's remarkable results with a diet consisting of whole plant foods that forbid oil extracts, seeds, and nuts suggest less to be best.

CHAPTER IV PROTEIN
Predicted Poison or Powerful Potion?

Protein is a nutrient with a positive and highly regarded reputation. Protein and muscle are terms used together favorably as though one without the other cannot exist. Because protein is chosen to nourish muscle growth it can do no harm, right? This chapter raises a legitimate question regarding the protein, whether it is a powerful life-giving potion or a poison that triggers compromised health resulting in disease.

Over the years, scientists have measured protein quality by how many grams of protein are required to attain growth from eating a specific food. The higher the weight-gain attributed to eating a food, the higher that food is rated. Dense muscle weight actually weighs 20% more than fat weight per cubic unit. Animal-source proteins typically are ranked higher than plant-source proteins quality when using the following rating scales: Protein Efficiency Ratio PER, Net Protein Utilization NPU, Biological Value BV, and Chemical Score CS:

Food	Protein Efficiency Ratio PER	Net Protein Utilization NPU	Biological Value BV	Chemical Score CS
Egg	4.2	1.00	0.99	1.00
Beef	2.4	0.80	0.74	0.80
Dairy	3.2	0.75	0.85	0.60
Fish	3.1	0.83	0.85	0.75
Rice	2.1	0.57	0.70	0.75
Corn	0.9	0.55	0.54	0.45
Wheat	1.6	0.52	0.64	0.59
ANIMAL FOODS AVERAGE 1.42 (PER/NPU/BV/CS)				
PLANT FOODS AVERAGE 1.10 (PER/NPU/BV/CS)[45]				

---

[45] Average Protein PER/NPU/BV/CS-score is 29% in favor of animal source foods egg, beef, dairy, and fish over rice, corn, and wheat.

The importance of protein in diet has been over-emphasized. The daily basic adult requirement for dietary protein ranges between 0.8 grams protein to 1.4 grams protein per kilogram body weight. Only in countries where severe starvation occurs is protein deficiency a factor in health issues. When humans starve due to lack of food for long periods of time, the probability of death increases when 40% of their original normal bodyweight is lost. Scientists report the relative risk of death by starvation increases after 20-60 days not eating.[46] Starvation causes a higher rate of loss in some tissue sites but less in others. Bodyweight fat loss can be as high as -97%, total body weight loss up to -40%, muscle mass loss -31%, blood loss -27%, bone loss -14%, but when heart muscle, nerve or brain tissue loss approach 3%, death by starvation occurs. Modern industrialized nations typically suffer more from excess weight gain virtually never from severe starvation, unless self-induced anorexia is imposed.

ANIMAL FOOD PROTEIN GROWTH MAY COMPROMISE HEALTH

Animal protein stimulates significant growth effect based on time and dose. Protein-induced growth effect may be associated with harmful effects on health.

---

[46] From Keys, Ancel, Joseph Brozek , Austin Henchel, Olaf Mickelson and Henry L. Taylor, (1950) *The Biology of Human Starvation.* Two Vols. Minneapolis: University of Minnesota Press.

Biological value (BV) is a measure of the proportion of protein absorbed from a food after digestion. BV is similar to PER, NPU, CS rating scale method. BV summarizes how readily a digested protein is synthesized into living cells. Proteins, unlike carbohydrates and fats, are the major source of nitrogen from the food chain. The average Biological value (BV) for protein score is 1.10 for plant food proteins and 1.42 for animal food proteins (29% higher in animal foods). The question here is how much relative nitrogen (from protein digested) is required? Should humans eat highest nitrogen-producing foods after their growth is attained? The gold standard for nitrogen-rich protein is human breast milk. It is the perfect food to promulgate growth when human growth rate is at its highest rate.

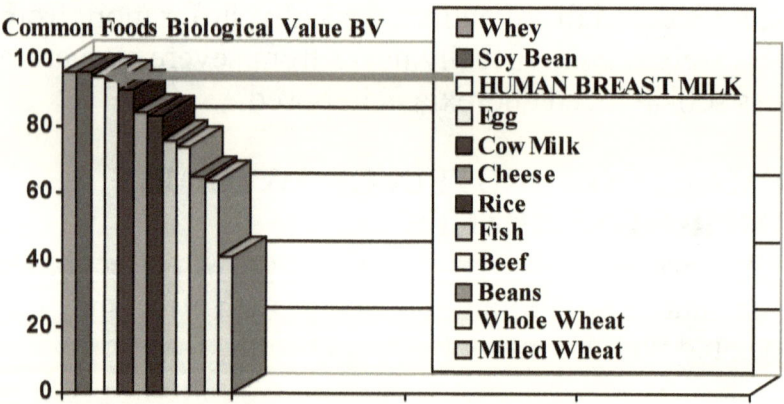

GROWTH RATE JUSTIFIES PROTEIN REQUIREMENT

A baby grows and enlarges at their most rapid rate during the first year of life. In 1-year, a newborn grows about 10 inches in length.

In the second year, growth slows to about 5 inches. By age seven, children are only growing only about 2 inches each year. Since human growth rate is highest the first 2-years of life, we may consider that nature's provision of human breast milk, is the model protein food for growth when it is at highest rate. Since human growth typically ceases after 20 years (+/-3-years), the dietary protein requirement (essential amino acids) is reduced. The protein (essential amino acids) units our body cannot make are isoleucine, leucine, valine, lysine, methionine, phenylalanine, threonine, tryptophan, and histidine. This following list shows milligram content of each essential amino acid gram weight in Human Breast Milk, Cow Milk, Soy, & Whey.

The essential amino acids EAA-profile produce a growth effect specific to the intended nursing offspring:

ESSENTIAL AMINO ACIDS MILLIGRAMS PER GRAM PROTEIN					
Amino Acid	Human Milk	Cow Milk	Soy	Whey	WHO [47] EAA
Isoleucine	54.55mg	60.35mg	49mg	54mg	20mg/kg
Leucine	92.50mg	97.91mg	82mg	89mg	39mg/kg
Valine	61.27mg	67.00mg	48mg	82mg	26mg/kg
Histidine	24.35mg	23.75mg	19mg	16mg	----------
Lysine	66.01mg	79.31mg	64mg	88mg	30mg/kg
Methionine	20.44mg	25.25mg	26mg	32mg	15mg/kg
Phenylalanine	44.67mg	48.40mg	38mg	32mg	25mg/kg
Threonine	44.67mg	45.08mg	38mg	65mg	15mg/kg
Tryptophan	16.52mg	14.16mg	14mg	22mg	4mg/kg
Totals	424.98mg	461.21mg	378mg	480mg	174mg/kg

---

[47] WHO-2001: Fürst P, Stehle P (1 June 2004). "What are the essential elements needed for the determination of amino acid requirements in humans?". J. Nutr. 134 (6 Suppl): 1558S–1565S. EAA, Essential amino acid requirements listed in mg/kg

The need to consume "essential amino acids" listed by WHO (2001) from the preceding table has been questioned by research showing that humans maintain nitrogen balance by consuming plant foods alone. This includes foods that lack one or more of the essential amino acids. Mike Anderson's review of this premise stated, "The first thing the human body does with a digested protein (complete with all the essential amino acids) is break it into pieces so it can mix and match specific amino acids for the body's specific needs at the time."[48] Research in humans shows subjects attained nitrogen balance after eating either corn alone, or potatoes alone, or rice alone. [49] The original requirement for the so-called "essential amino acids" was based on rats growth rate. This may be the source of our problem with eating too much protein. Humans do not have the same protein requirement as either rats or cows! Since growth is highest for all species after birth during pre-weaning years, the nutrient profile of mother's milk is nutrient species-specific. Comparing human and cow milk shows remarkably different properties and effects:

WHAT ARE THE DIFFERENCES BETWEEN HUMAN MILK & COW MILK? [50]

---

[48] Healing Cancer from the inside out. www.RaveDiet.com April 2009. p135.

[49] Kofrányi E, Jekat F, Müller-Wecker H. The determination of the biological value of dietary proteins. XVI. The minimum protein requirement of humans, tested with mixtures of whole egg plus potato and maize plus beans. Hoppe Seylers Z Physiol Chem. 1970 Dec;351(12):1485-93; Clark HE, Malzer JL, Onderka HM, Howe JM, Moon W. Nitrogen balances of adult human subjects fed combinations of wheat, beans, corn, milk, and rice. Am J Clin Nutr. 1973 Jul;26(7):702-6; Edwards CH, Booker LK, Rumph CH, Wright WG, Ganapathy SN. Utilization of wheat by adult man: nitrogen metabolism, plasma amino acids and lipids. Am J Clin Nutr. 1971 Feb;24(2):181-93; Clark HE, Howe JM, Lee CJ. Nitrogen retention of adult human subjects fed a high protein rice. Am J Clin Nutr. 1971 Mar;24(3):324-8; Kies C, Williams E, Fox HM. Determination of first limiting nitrogenous factor in corn protein for nitrogen retention in human adults. J Nutr. 1965 Aug;86:3.

Some of the effects and ingredients of nursed milks in the intended offspring are listed below:

Macronutrient Content	Human Milk	Cow Milk
Total Milk calories nursed per 1-ounce weight gain	1000 k/cal = 1-ounce weight gain	350 k/cal = 1-ounce weight gain
Calories per fluid ounce	21.4 k/cal	18.75 k/cal
Macronutrient profile [51]	6% protein 39% carbohydrates 55% fat	21% protein 30% carbohydrates 49% fat
Weight Gain Calories per pound	16,000 calories Human Milk generates one lb weight gain [52]	5,600 calories Cow Milk in calf generates one lb weight gain [53]

Protein & Micronutrient Content *(G/100 ML)*	Human Milk	Cow Milk
PROTEIN (G/100 ML) total	1.1	3.3
Casein 0.4 *(G/100 ML)*	0.3	2.5
alpha-lactalbumin	0.3	0.1
Lactoferrin	0.2	trace
IgA	0.1	0.003
IgG	0.001	0.06
Lysozyme	0.05	trace
Serum Albumin	0.05	0.03
ß-lactoglobulin	-	0.3
Fat - total (g/100 ml)	4.2	3.8
Fatty acids £ 8C (%)	trace	6
Polyunsaturated fatty acids (%)	14	3
Carbohydrate Lactose (g/100 ml)	7.0	4.8
Carbohydrates (g/100 ml) Oligosaccharides	0.5	0.005
Calcium *(G/100 ML)*	0.030	0.125
Phosphorus *(G/100 ML)*	0.014	0.093
Sodium *MG/100 ML)*	0.015	0.047
Potassium *(G/100 ML)*	0.055	0.155
Chlorine *(G/100 ML)*	0.043	0.103

50 Constituents of human milk, Ann Prentice,
http://www.unu.edu/unupress/food/8F174e/8F174E04.htm
51 Computed by First Data Bank Nutritionist IV Dietary Analysis software program.
52 Human breast milk requires 286% more calories to generate one-pound body weight in humans.
53 Cows' milk requires 35% less total calories to generate one-pound growth in a calf. Weight gain in calves is nearly triple that observed in human infants.

GROWTH EFFECTS FROM COW MILK & HUMAN MILK DIFFER All the nutrients required for a human infant's growth compared to a cow-calf growth prior to weaning differ significantly. No responsible rationale supports that one species should consume milk met for another species each with differing growth rates. Cow's milk has a completely different macronutrient and micronutrient structure than human breast milk. Cow's milk is designed to support the growth pattern of a cow, while human milk is designed to support growth pattern of a human. The rate of growth when a cow consumes cow's milk or a human consumes human milk per pound weight gain differs remarkably.[43] [44] The essential amino acids profile differs significantly between human breast milk and cow's milk. A calf gains 1-pound weight nursing only 5,600 calories cow milk, while a human baby and the same stage of life must consume 16,000 calories of mom's breast milk to gain the same 1-pound body weight. Given a calf has a different genetic makeup causing weight gains faster than a human, yet when human infants consume cow's milk, they actually gain weight much faster on less calories as compared with nursing human breast milk. Because 21% of the cow milk calories are proteins designed to stimulate rapid calf growth as compared to 6% protein in human breast milk, cow milk's higher protein content is shown to be the activating trigger that causes excessive growth gain in humans.

Researchers concluded that the more cow milk children consumed, the more weight they gained, and conversely the less cow milk they consumed, the less weight they gained: [54]

---

[54] Although the magnitudes of our estimated dietary effects (on 1-year BMI change) were small, they may accumulate over time and become clinically important if high intakes

Children who consumed higher total milk intake experienced larger weight gains.

Children who drank more 1% or skim milk had larger weight gains than those who drank smaller amounts of 1% or skim milk.

Dietary calcium intake was positively correlated with weight gain.

Dairy fat was not correlated with weight gain.

All micronutrients calcium, potassium, sodium, chlorine, and phosphorous were 200-600% higher in cow's milk than human breast milk. The total calories are higher in human breast milk than cow's milk. Fat and carbohydrate calories are higher in human breast milk than cow's milk. The only macronutrient that is higher in cow's milk than human breast milk is protein. Protein per unit of milk is +300% higher in cow's milk than human breast milk. Perhaps it is protein excess that causes humans to gain weight faster nursing cow's milk than human breast milk. This suggests that dietary protein volume (how much protein) is a prominent factor-effecting rate of growth with implications for health or disease.

PROTEIN GROWTH EFFECT QUESTIONED
The average rating scale[55] for protein growth gain from animal foods is 1.42 while plant food protein is 1.10, or 29%.

---

persist for multiple years (Berkey et al., 2005).
[55] Protein Efficiency Ratio PER, Net Protein Utilization NPU, Biological Value BV, and Chemical Score CS listed on page 27.

The growth-gain effect from consuming "complete/quality" proteins is now in question. Cornell nutrition scientist, T. Colin Campbell concluded "Protein-induced rapid growth in children is not necessarily a desirable end." [56]

Specific animal research show when rats are exposed to a carcinogen (Aflatoxin) with 20% of their protein calories from milk, grew tumors, while those eating only 5% did not grow tumors.[57] By decreasing the amount of milk protein, researchers found they could turn off carcinogen binding effect that causes cancers. [58]

DIETARY PROTEIN CARCINOGEN
AFLATOXIN-INDUCED LIVER CANCE
(Campbell 1989)

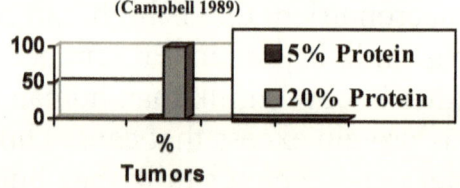

[56] Lecture TCC502 eCornell Plant Food Certificate Course, By permission, courtesy of Dr. T. Colin Campbell @: http://www.tcolincampbell.org/
[57] Madhavan TV, Gopalan C. The effect of dietary protein on carcinogenesis of aflatoxin. Arch Pathol. 1968 Feb;85(2):133-7.
[58] Campbell TC. "Influence of nutrition on metabolism of carcinogens (Martha Maso's Honors Thesis)". Adv. Nutr. Res. 2(1979):29-55.

The question, "Is excess dietary protein a stimulant associated with abnormal cancer cell production?" Preneoplastic Foci cells are pre-cancer cell growths destined to form tumors. Youngman and Campbell also confirmed this finding that a combination of a high intake 20% animal protein (cow milk) with carcinogen exposure (Aflatoxin) significantly increased pre-cancer Foci cell growth, while a low intake 5% of this protein at the same rate of carcinogen exposure did not result in an increased cell growth: [59] [60]

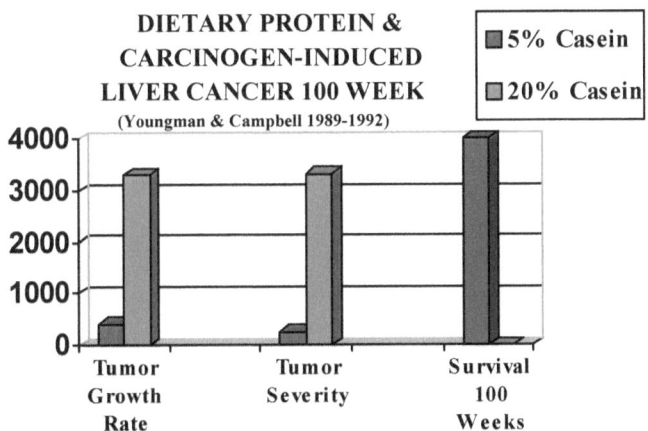

HOW MUCH CARCINOGEN CAUSES CANCER?
The typical carcinogen dose needed to cause cancer in an animal research studies is huge, more than humans are typically exposed to on a day-by-day basis.

[59] Youngman LD, Campbell TC. High protein intake promotes the growth of hepatic in Fischer #344 rats: evidence that early remodeled foci retain the potential for future growth. J Nutr. 1991 Sep;121(9):1454-61.
[60] Youngman LD, Campbell TC. Inhibition of aflatoxin B1-induced gamma-glutamyltranspeptidase positive (GGT+) hepatic preneoplastic foci and tumors by low protein diets: evidence that altered GGT+ foci indicate neoplastic potential. Carcinogenesis. 1992 Sep;13(9):1607-13.

The chart, "HUMAN COMPARED TO ANIMAL RESEARCH CARCINOGEN EXPOSURE," illustrates probability of cancer based on exposure rates; please note the amount research animals receive compared to what human environmental exposure.

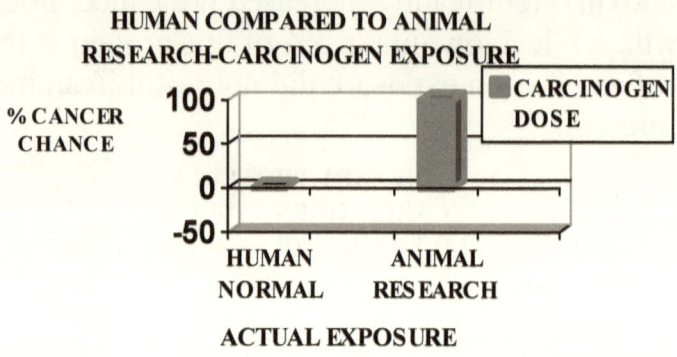

The typical daily human carcinogen exposure is far less than the amounts consumed by animals in research projects. For a particular carcinogen to cause cancer in animals, it must be consumed at an extraordinarily high dose. Nitrosamine, for example, was given to rats in order to produce precancerous Foci cells. How much nitrosamine in human terms would it take to cause cancer? Nitrosamine in tiny amounts is commonly found in the lunchmeat, bologna. Eating a 1-pound bologna sandwich produces only 1/270000th of a single dose needed to induce cancers in rats.

A human would have to eat 270,000 bologna sandwiches in order to be exposed to the same amount of nitrosamine that triggers cancer cell activity in rats. Since such an unlikely carcinogen dose ever occurs to humans, why is cancer so prevalent in our culture? A hypothetical model suggests that each carcinogen requires a specific trigger to provoke DNA-mutation effects. Such effects are increased following exposure to dangerous substances, such as virus, bacteria, or radiation.

When scientists fed protein to rats exposed to toxic levels of a common carcinogen, they found when the rats ate more protein than their bodies required above 10% of their body need, the rate of precursor cancer cells (foci) increased. [61] However, at 10% or less of their total calories from the same milk protein, foci cancer cell production was reduced.

They discovered they could turn on or turn off the precursor cancer cell production simply by turning down the amount of animal source dietary protein fed to carcinogen-exposed rats. Too much protein above what the rats required had a triggering effect increasing cancer cell production. This evidence states that what we eat may be more of the cause of cancers than to what amount of carcinogen we are exposed.

---

[61] Dunaif GE, Campbell TC. Dietary protein level and aflatoxin B1-induced preneoplastic hepatic lesions in the rat. J Nutr. 1987 Jul;117(7):1298-302.

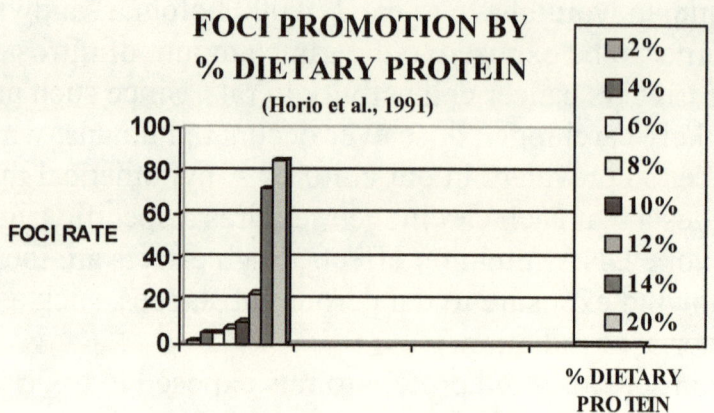

FOCI PROMOTION BY % DIETARY PROTEIN
(Horio et al., 1991)

FOCI RATE

% DIETARY PROTEIN

- □ 2%
- ■ 4%
- □ 6%
- □ 8%
- ■ 10%
- ■ 12%
- ■ 14%
- □ 20%

Horio F, Youngman LD, Bell RC, Campbell TC. Thermogenesis, low-protein diets, and decreased development of AFB1-induced preneoplastic foci in rat liver. Nutr Cancer. 1991;16(1):31-41.

WHAT KIND OF PROTEIN TRIGGERS CARCINOGEN-INDUCED CANCER?

Researchers sought to identify the protein triggering mechanisms more clearly. They found that the type of protein fed to the rats increased precursor foci-cancer cells. They kept the carcinogen-exposure rate constant, but fed different types of protein foods, cow milk protein or plant proteins from wheat gluten or soy: [62]

---

[62] Schulsinger DA, Root MM, Campbell TC. Effect of dietary protein quality on development of aflatoxin B1-induced hepatic preneoplastic lesions. J Natl Cancer Inst. 1989 Aug 16;81(16):1241-5.

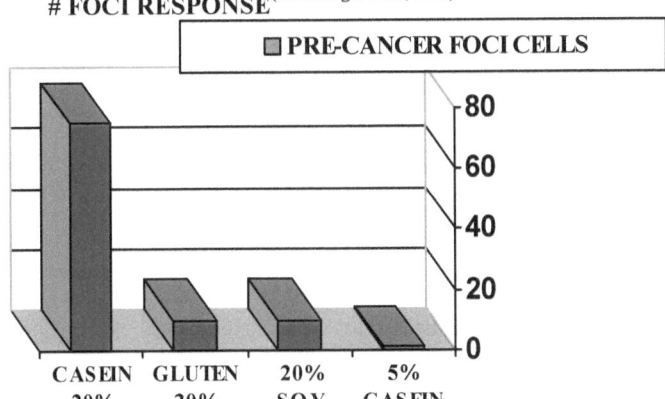

PROTEIN FOOD INCREASE
FOCI RESPONSE (Schulsinger et al., 1989)

The type of protein provoking precursor cancer cell production increased when carcinogen-exposed animals consumed animal sourced milk protein 20%. However, when animals consumed plant food proteins, such as gluten or soy at the same 20% of their total calories, foci cell growths were significantly less. Rat and human protein requirements are similar. Human protein requirements never exceed 10% of the total calories consumed. For example, human breast milk contains only 5% of its calories as protein. The protein supplied by human breast milk supports infant growth during our highest growth rate. If we consume more protein than needed is this harmful to health? Currently the average protein consumed in America ranges between 15-16%, or around 300-320 protein calories out of every 2000 calories intake. On average, this can be calculated as 23 gallons milk, 30 pounds of cheese, and 23 pounds of ice cream per year. That is a lot of cow milk protein when one considers it is the milk intended for another species!

Mutant cancers can be caused by a genetic disorder and may be aggressively activated by diet choices. Researchers fed 6%, 14%, and 22% protein calories from the cow milk, to two strains of hepatitis HBV-infected transgenic mice. [63] A genetic defect was activated resulting in an increased rate of liver cancer. As the percents of dietary cow milk protein increased, so did the rate of gene-expressed HBV-liver cancers:

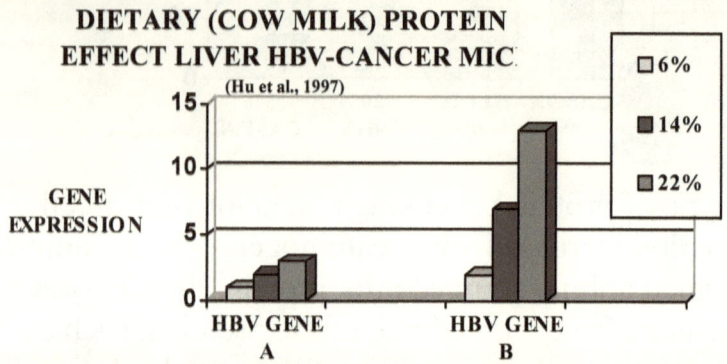

Hu J. et al., "Repression of Hepatitis B virus (HBV)transgene and HBV-induced liver injury by low protein diet." Oncogene 15 (1997):2795-2801.

When 10% or less of the calories consumed from cow milk, there was significantly less cancer formation in both transgenic and carcinogen-exposed animals. Once the percent of protein calories from cow milk exceeded 10%, the rate of cancer increased proportionately. [64]

The Horio et al., graph further illustrates this effect further: [65]

---

[63] Hu JF, Cheng Z, Chisari FV, Vu TH, Hoffman AR, Campbell TC. Repression of hepatitis B virus (HBV) transgene and HBV-induced liver injury by low protein diet. Oncogene. 1997 Dec 4;15(23):2795-801.
[64] Dunaif GE, Campbell TC. Dietary protein level and aflatoxin B1-induced preneoplastic hepatic lesions in the rat. J Nutr. 1987 Jul;117(7):1298-302.
[65] Horio F, Youngman LD, Bell RC, Campbell TC. Thermogenesis, low-protein diets, and decreased development of AFB1-induced preneoplastic foci in rat liver. Nutr Cancer.

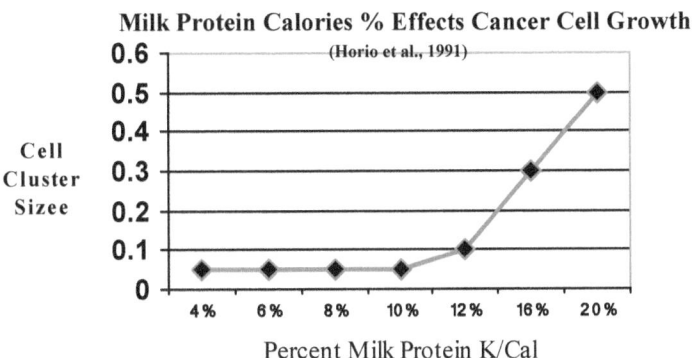

Milk Protein Calories % Effects Cancer Cell Growth
(Horio et al., 1991)

Cell Cluster Sizee

Percent Milk Protein K/Cal

IS MEAT PROTEIN HARMFUL?

The term "Meat Protein" includes all forms of meat, whether high or low in harmful substances such as saturated fat and cholesterol. Harmful effects associated with eating meats of a living creature may be based on the associated rate of kidney stone formations. The more beef, fish, and poultry consumed, the greater the risk of kidney stones. The suspected mechanism is urinary calcium loss from a high renal acid load, a direct result from eating meat.

Robertson reported that it takes eating only 20-grams meat to increase the rate of kidney stone formation. [66] A Big-Mac Hamburger contains 25-grams of animal protein, more than enough to discharge kidney stones in persons so predisposed. Most Americans are consuming from 70-100 grams protein from animal origins every day!

1991;16(1):31-41.
[66] Robertson WG, Peacock M, and Hodgkinson A. "Dietary changes and in the incidence of urinary calculi in the UK between 1958 and 1976." Chron. Dis. 32 (1979): 469-476.

IS MEAT HARMFUL?

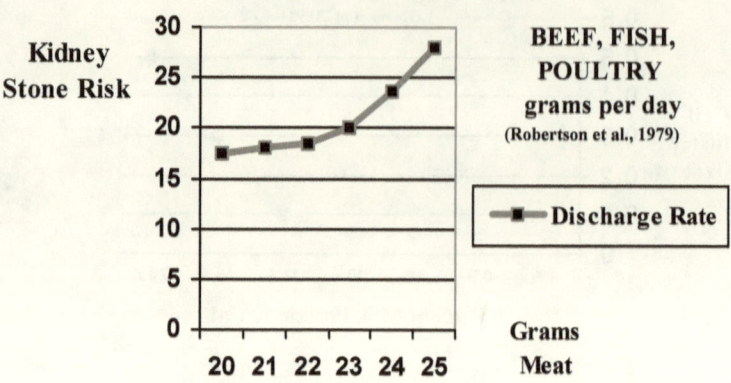

A basic biochemistry principle (mechanism) suggests animal protein plays a prominent role in the development of disease by negatively impacting the contribution of vitamin D for preventing disease. Numerous studies point a critical finger naming animal source meats and milk as prominent associations with disease. Scientists reported a link between a hormone, Insulin-like Growth Factor-1, shown to boost division of cell growth in men diagnosed with prostate cancer.

Previous studies showed that levels of this hormone are higher in men who eat excessive amounts of meat, cheese, milk, and butter. By contrast, vegetarians have low Insulin-like Growth Factor-1 levels. [67] Data from another study also confirms there is a modest association of colorectal cancer risk with elevated serum IGF-I. [68] Researchers showed that only a 5% increase in energy in dietary fat intake from meat was associated with a 21% increase in the likelihood of having one additional CVD risk factor. Such findings support the hypothesis that consumption of fat from meat or its byproduct increase CVD risk factors among the elderly. [69] High protein intake from meat or fish is associated with an increased risk of incident IBD in French middle-aged women. [70]

T. Colin Campbell clearly stated, "Animal food (through its protein and saturated fat content) raises the risk of Type I diabetes, Lupus, rheumatoid arthritis, and MS." [71] The higher the amount of dairy milk consumed, the higher the rate of Type 1 diabetes [72] and Multiple Sclerosis MS [73]. The higher the amount of dairy milk consumed, the higher the risk of osteoporosis.[60][61]

This chart following demonstrates these findings:

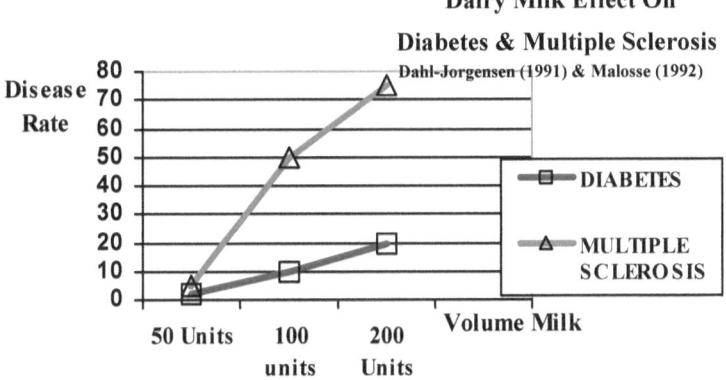

Dairy Milk Effect On Diabetes & Multiple Sclerosis

[67] Roddam AW, et al., Insulin-like growth factors, their binding proteins, and prostate cancer risk: analysis of individual patient data from 12 prospective studies. Ann Intern Med. 2008 Oct 7;149(7):461-71, W83-8.

[68] Rinaldi S, et al., Serum levels of IGF-I, IGFBP-3 and colorectal cancer risk: results from the EPIC cohort, plus a meta-analysis of prospective studies. Int J Cancer. 2010 Apr 1;126(7):1702-15.

[69] Polychronopoulos E, et al., Dietary meat fats and burden of cardiovascular disease risk factors, in the elderly: a report from the MEDIS study. Lipids Health Dis. 2010 Mar 18;9:30.

[70] Jantchou P, Morois S, Clavel-Chapelon F, Boutron-Ruault MC, Carbonnel F. Animal Protein Intake and Risk of Inflammatory Bowel Disease: The E3N Prospective Study. Am J Gastroenterol. 2010 May 11.

[71] Lecture TCC502 Dr. T. Colin Campbell in eCornell Plant Food Certificate Course @: http://www.ecornell.com/certificate-programs/personal-interest-training/certificate-in-plant-based-nutrition-certificate/crt/TCCC01

[72] Dahl-Jorgensen K, Joner G, and Hanssen KF. "Relationship between cow's milk consumption and incidence of IDDM in childhood." Diabetes Care 14 (1991): 1081-1085.

[73] Malosse D, Perron H, Sasco A, et al. "Correlation between milk and dairy product consumption and multiple sclerosis prevalence: a worldwide study." Neuroepidemiology 11 (1992): 304-312.

The higher the consumption of animal protein correlates to a higher consumption of calcium, typically from a higher consumption of dairy milk that increases the risk of osteoporosis. Scientists assessed data from 33 countries and concluded that as vegetable to animal protein ratio increases, the rate of bone fractures dramatically decreases. [74] (In other words, the people ate more vegetable protein than animal protein experienced a lower rate of bone fractures). Women with the highest ratio of animal protein to plant protein had 3.7 times more bone fractures than the women consuming the lowest ratio. Animal protein tends to produce more acid in both the blood and the urine. Eating any animal meats or cow milk byproducts raises urinary loss of calcium. Acid in the blood stream or urine pulls calcium out of the bones and raises the risk of osteoporosis or bone fractures.

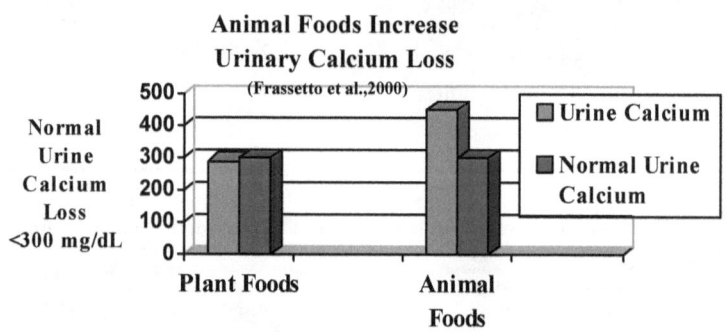

Since Type I Diabetes, Lupus, Rheumatoid Arthritis, Osteoporosis, and MS are influenced by a food's structure effecting pH in the body, what are the structural composite differences between animal foods and plant foods?

[74] Frassetto LA, Todd KM, Morris C, Jr., et al. "World incidence of hip fracture in elderly women relation to consumption of animal and vegetable foods." J. Gerentology 55 (2000): M585-M592.

MACRONUTRIENT STRUCTURAL DIFFERENCES IN ANIMAL FOODS & PLANT FOODS

The macronutrient profile of animal-foods compared to plant-foods shows that their protein, carbohydrate, fat, and renal acid load ^{pH} values differ significantly. [75] The total calories, cholesterol, and renal acid load are remarkably in less plant foods than in animal- foods:

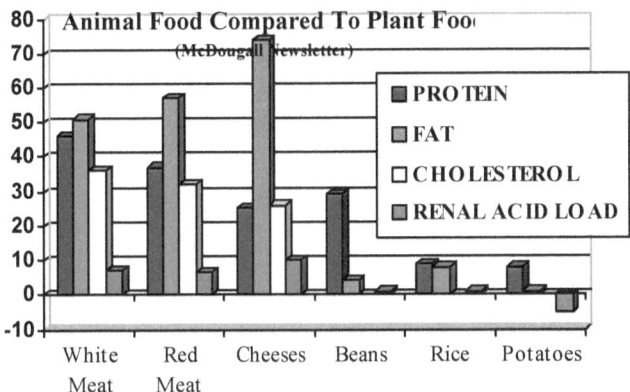

WHERE DO YOU GET YOUR PROTEIN IF YOU EAT ONLY PLANT FOODS?

People often ask plant food eaters, "Where do you get your protein?" Protein digested foods must broken apart into amino acids. The amino acids are absorbed from the small intestines, carried to the liver for processing later into the blood circulation. Amino acids are distributed to the specific body tissues where they are needed. The required protein to maintain nitrogen balance is only 0.36 grams protein per pound body weight.

---

[75] McDougall Newsletter at http://www.drmcdougall.com

With increasing calorie expenditure, such as prolonged exercise or physical work, the requirement may increase up to 0.63 grams protein per pound body weight. Consuming more than 0.36-0.63 grams protein per pound body weight may raise circulating urea and/or nitrogen excess high enough to induce premature fatigue and unwanted, unnecessary gain in Body Mass Index. [76]

The Recommended Daily Allowance (RDA) is 10-15% of calories as protein from diet. A number of whole plant foods contain high quality protein ranging from 14%-40% for easily meeting the protein required:

PLANT FOOD	Protein grams/100 grams Food
Spinach	40.000
Tempeh Soy-Fermented	40.000
Soybeans	36.490
Broccoli	33.000
Asparagus	31.000
Winged beans, mature seeds, raw	29.650
Lentils, mature seeds, raw	28.060
Cauliflower	27.000
Broadbeans (fava beans)	26.120
Brussels Sprouts	26.000
Beans, kidney, royal red, mature seeds, raw	25.330
Yardlong beans, mature seeds, raw	24.330
Mung beans, mature seeds, raw	23.860
Beans, white, mature seeds, raw	23.360
Beans, cranberry (roman)	23.030
Kale	23.000
Mothbeans, mature seeds, raw	22.940
Beans, navy, mature seeds, raw	22.330
Beans, yellow, mature seeds, raw	22.000
Beans, great northern, mature seeds, raw	21.860
Beans, black, mature seeds, raw	21.600
Lima beans, large, mature seeds, raw	21.460
Beans, small white, mature seeds, raw	21.110
PLANT FOOD	Protein grams/100 grams Food

[76] Hermanussen M., Nutritional protein intake is associated with body mass index in young adolescents. Georgian Med News. 2008 Mar;(156):84-8.

Beans, pink, mature seeds, raw	20.960
Beans, pinto, mature seeds, raw	20.880
Beans, adzuki, mature seeds, raw	19.870
Flax seed	19.500
Chickpeas (garbanzo beans)	19.300
Oats	16.890
Tofu, raw, firm	15.780
Cabbage	15.000
Tomatoes	14.110
Quinoa	14.100
Beets	13.000

The average weight of total foods (taken from dietary analysis performed on a variety of subjects between 1996-2010) ranges to as little as 1200 grams to as much as 3400 grams total food weight per day. Let's examine this by example; if each of person ate only 100 grams of 10 lowest protein plant foods for a totaling 1000-grams food/day (from adzuki beans, pinto beans, garbanzo beans, oats, tofu, cabbage, tomatoes, quinoa, beets, kale), they would consume enough protein. Note: the weight of these 10 foods is less than the lowest total food weight from any diets I have previously analyzed in 14 years.

A computerized dietary analysis of 10-foods[77] produce 1445 calories with 76-grams protein, more than enough required protein for a 209 lb person! Though eating 1445 calories would not satisfy the appetite of the typical average American who eats over 1980 calories average per day, but the protein amount would easily smeat the daily RDA required amount.

---

[77] First Data Bank Nutritionist Pro IV Dietary Analysis of 100 grams each food, 6-18-2010 (adzuki beans, pinto beans, garbanzo beans, oats, tofu, cabbage, tomatoes, quinoa, beets, kale) 1000 grams total, 1445 k/cal, 20% protein, 69% carbohydrate, 11 % fat.

The point is that plant foods do contain adequate high quality, easily digestible protein without the unnecessary saturated fats, cholesterol, and harmful toxic substances found higher in the food chain from animal-sources red meat, milk, poultry, or fish.

The average woman needs only 30 grams protein per day, the average man needs around 40 grams per day to maintain positive nitrogen balance. Eating 2000 calories from only oats, would provide 82 grams of protein, 2000 calories of corn provides 53 grams protein, even eating 2000 calories of watermelon, would provide 40 grams protein. The healthy effect from eating plant foods compared to the toxic effects associated with eating animal proteins the following are concluded:

Conclusions:
1. Rating protein quality sets a false standard for "essential amino acids" required for human health.
2. Protein deficiency in humans occurs only during severe starvation and weight loss.
3. Protein requirements for adults is 10% or less of total bodyweight sustaining calories.
4. Growth effects from all animal foods proteins may compromise health.
5. Growth effects from plant food proteins do not compromise health.
6. Human breast milk is the gold standard for human protein requirements.
7. Cow milk is the gold standard for calf protein requirement.
8. Cow milk protein causes an increased rate of weight gain in humans.

9. Cow milk providing between 10-20% of the total protein calories stimulates cancer cell production in carcinogen-exposed rats.
10. Plant food proteins providing 20% of the total calories do not stimulate cancer cell production in carcinogen-exposed rats.
11. Cow milk consumed at 6-20% percent of protein of total calories increases rate of genetic-associated cancers in HBV-infected mice. The higher the %-protein, the higher the cancer growth rate gene expression.
12. Animal meat consumption above 20-grams inhibits normal calcium metabolism and increases the risk of kidney stone formation. This has been associated with serious consequences to vitamin D and Calcium metabolism resulting in disease progression.
13. Animal milk or meats consumption raises the risk of Type I diabetes, Lupus, rheumatoid arthritis, osteoporosis, and MS.
14. The macronutrient profile of animal compared to plant foods rules in favor of plant foods due their lower calorie, lower cholesterol, and a lower renal acid load effects.
15. There is no human physiological requirement for animal-protein calories.

PRACTICAL APPLICATIONS PROTEIN - What do I do?

➤ Remove all dairy milk calories from your diet.
➤ Remove all meats or meat byproducts from your diet.
➤ Remove all packaged-processed foods from your diet.
➤ Remove all extracted oils, seeds, nuts, and foods with high fat content from diet.

- Consume only proteins from whole plant foods.
- Consume only fats in whole plant foods, never extract forms.
- Consume only carbohydrates in whole plant foods.
- Expect cholesterol to significantly decrease within 14-days initiating a whole plant food diet. Any variation from whole plant lifestyle, including transitory "Whole plant foods" substitutes will inhibit progress toward reduced cholesterol levels.
- Expect blood sugar levels to significantly decrease within 14-days application of a whole plant food diet. Any variation from Whole Plant Foods including transitory substitutes for "Whole Plant Foods" will inhibit progress toward lowering blood sugar levels.
- Expect body fat loss within 21-40-days application of a whole plant food diet.
- Expect energy and cognitive levels to increase within 21-days application of a whole plant food diet.
- Expect cravings increase between start and up to 40-days after application of a whole plant food diet.
- Cravings resolution may require up to 90-days application of a whole plant food diet.
- Expect cravings to change toward whole plant foods, taste preferences to require as long as 40-90 days after application of a whole plant food diet.
- Abstained foods removed from living quarters will assist taste and cravings control. "If it is in the house, it will likely find its way into the mouth." Refuse access to, abstain from and remove all animal-sourced foods.
- Reduce appetite cravings by hydrating 30-minutes prior to eating; eating high fiber fruits or vegetables prior to eating calorie-dense foods will curb appetite remarkably.

➢ Consume an adequate protein minimum of 0.36 grams protein per pound body weight per day to maintain nitrogen balance.
➢ Plant food protein adequately replenishes required protein. Fatigue is a sign of deficient protein intake and excess amounts.
➢ Consume no more than 0.63 grams protein per pound body weight per day.
➢ Calorie intake from plant foods ranging between 1400-1900 k/cal per day easily meets the protein requirement for a 210 lb person.

CHAPTER V CARBOHYDRATES
Phytonutrient Glucose Control

The human body's energy currency is glucose. Glucose levels from a dietary health perspective must be controlled. Carbohydrates stored make up only 1% of human body weight, thus humans do not need copious amounts of carbohydrates to maintain health. In fact too much of this nutrient may stimulate a high glycemic effect on blood sugar causing our appetite to eat more than needed. Herein lies the problem, if a carbohydrate feeding raises blood sugars too high or too fast, it may not only fail to satisfy our desires, it may spike cravings to eat more sweet-tasting sugars than necessary. Conversely, complex carbohydrates encased in whole plant food fibers (cellulose) do not raise blood sugar rapidly, and tend to fill and satisfy within an hour after consumed. Soluble complex carbohydrates eventually break down into glucose for energy conversion, or to be stored as either glycogen or body fat. Glycogen is stored in the liver to maintain normal blood sugar levels or in the muscles, where it can be withdrawn to generate energy for aerobic exercise. When muscle glycogen stores are full, any excess carbohydrate calories are converted into body fat, triglycerides, or cholesterol. Avoiding eating too much of a macronutrient that stimulates appetite must be controlled.

Excessive amounts of calorie-dense carbohydrates, rich in processed simple sugars, low in fiber, and antioxidant-poor have been associated with several health issues such as insulin resistance, diabetes, cardiovascular diseases, and cancers. Conversely, health-enhancing complex carbohydrates contain modest amounts of simple sugars, high in fiber, calorie-sparse, fluid-rich, and are high in antioxidants.

This is a description of whole, unprocessed plant foods. Generally speaking, plant foods raise blood glucose slowly. The measure of a digested food's effect on blood sugar level is called glycemic index (GI). Carbohydrates that digest quickly and release glucose rapidly into the bloodstream are high glycemic index carbohydrates, while those that break down slowly, releasing glucose gradually into the bloodstream, are low glycemic index. The lower glycemic index foods result in a lower insulin response. This effect is associated with healthy blood glucose and blood lipid control. Too much sugar in the blood stream repeated year after year is associated with diseases and premature death. Countries consuming the most plant foods also consumed the most complex carbohydrates and the least fat. This effect from their diet resulted in the lowest rate of diabetes death. Those countries consuming the most fat and the least plant food carbohydrates had the highest rate of diabetes death.

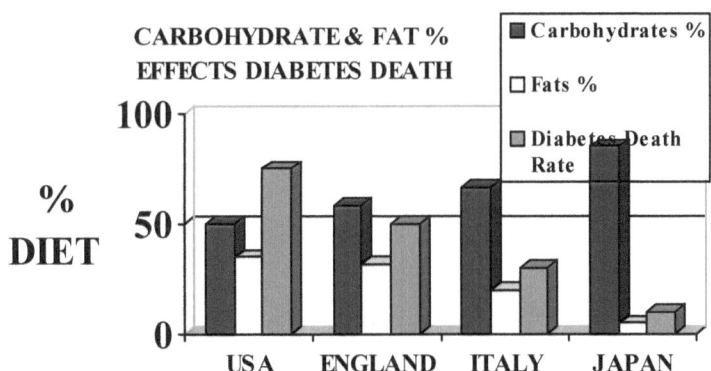

Blood glucose is controlled when fiber-rich whole plant foods are consumed. Fruits and vegetables produce a low glycemic effect because of their soluble fiber, insoluble fiber, and antioxidant content. The importance of dietary fiber volume cannot be overemphasized. The average fiber intake in the USA is 11-grams per day[78], well short of the 25-30 grams recommended each day. Whole, unrefined plant foods' higher soluble and insoluble fiber content with unrefined complex carbohydrates do not spike blood sugar nearly as high as refined, processed simple sugars. Whole plant foods have been linked with favorable lipoprotein profiles and reduced coronary heart disease risk. Persons eating whole plant foods typically consume double the fiber compared to those not eating whole plant foods. [79] Soluble fiber found in legumes, fruits, and vegetables lower plasma cholesterol.[80] Fruit, vegetables, leafy greens, and legumes also contain folic acid known to lower homocysteine. Elevated homocysteine is associated with increased risk of heart disease.[81] Whole plant foods, in their natural unprocessed form, contain a number of known and unknown phytonutrients that will reduce the onset of diseases common to industrialized nations' dietary foods whose phytonutrients have been removed.

How much and what are the best whole food carbohydrates?

Carbohydrate foods containing insoluble and soluble fiber help create a low glycemic effect on blood sugar concentrations.

---

[78] Lanza, E, Jones, DY, Block, G, Kessler, L Dietary fiber intake in the US population Am J Clin Nutr 1987 46: 790-797

[79] Ibid.

[80] Council on Scientific Affairs: Dietary fiber and health. JAMA 262: 542–546, 1989.

[81] Makoff R, Dwyer J, Rocco MV: Folic acid, pyridoxine, cobalamin, and homocysteine and their relationship to cardiovascular disease in end-stage renal disease. J Renal Nutr 6: 2–11, 1996.

The best food sources of soluble fiber are oatmeal, oatbran, legumes, beans, dried peas, lentils, apples, pears, strawberries, & blueberries. The best sources of insoluble fiber are whole wheat bread, barley, couscous, brown rice, bulgur, whole grain breakfast cereals, wheat bran, carrots, cucumbers, zucchini & celery. High soluble/insoluble fiber foods are associated with a reduced risk of hemorrhoids, homocysteine, blood pressure, ischemic heart disease, constipation, diverticulosis, gallstones, diarrhea, irritable bowel syndrome, colon cancer, (non-hodgkin's) lymphomas, prostate cancer, elevated blood sugar, elevated serum cholesterol, elevated triglycerides, diabetes mellitus type II, insulin resistance, and obesity. Human total required carbohydrates is 75-150 grams per day; however, the average person living in western nations ranges between 250-400 grams per day! We eat too much processed refined carbohydrates that elevate blood sugar, elevated blood fat, including excess weight gain. Researchers concluded, "Increasing intakes of refined carbohydrate (corn syrup) concomitant with decreasing intakes of fiber paralleled the upward trend in the prevalence of type 2 diabetes observed in the United States during the 20th century." [82]

As fiber and unrefined complex carbohydrates from whole plant foods decreased, refined simple sugar increased. Not only are Americans eating too much carbohydrate, they are eating the refined processed forms that are known to compromise healthy blood sugar and lipid fractions.

---

[82] Gross LS, Li L, Ford ES, Liu S. Increased consumption of refined carbohydrates and the epidemic of type 2 diabetes in the United States: an ecologic assessment. Am J Clin Nutr. 2004 May;79(5):774-9.

A health-enhancing diet should contain 50-55% of the total calories from complex carbohydrates, (long-chain polysaccharides), specifically those with a high-fiber, low glycemic index with no more than 15% simple sugar. The recommended adequate daily intake of (minimum) dietary fiber is 21-25 grams for adult women and 30-38 grams per day for adult men. Our current average daily fiber intake for women is 13-15 grams and for men is 17-19 grams per day. If both men and women's fiber intake exceeded 30 grams per day, health profile would improve dramatically. This low fiber intake permits harmful levels of food toxins, fats, cholesterols, and sugars to invade circulation resulting in compromised health. If 3/4th of our calories come from vegetables, fruits, whole grains and beans, harmful blood fats, excessive blood sugar, and destructive toxins will be dramatically reduced. Fiber is nearly absent from packaged, processed foods. The milling of grains, peeling of fruits and vegetables removes most of the natural plant fibers. Soft drinks, sweetened-processed breakfast cereals, candy, fruit drinks, and dairy byproducts are low-fiber foods that contain excessive amounts of refined simple sugar. The total intake of processed, refined sugars must be strictly limited to no more than 15% of total carbohydrate calories.

What are the top fiber food sources? Ground flaxseeds and psyllium husks are two supplements that can be added to whole grain cereals, salads, or other foods. Wheat bran, oat bran, kale, asparagus, all sorts of beans such as white beans, pinto beans, lima beans, and lentils have excellent ratio providing both soluble and insoluble fiber content.

HIGH FIBER CARBOHYDRATE FOODS LIST

HIGH FIBER CARBOHYDRATE PREFERRED FOODS [83]			
(Highest to lowest sources in grams per 100 grams)			
Food Source	Total Fiber	Soluble Fiber	Insoluble Fiber
Wheat Bran	46.6	3.6	43
Flax Seeds	32.0	10.5	22
Oat Bran	30.3	15.3	15
White Beans	27.6	11.6	16
Pinto Beans	27.2	8.2	19
Kale	25.9	5.9	20
Lima Beans	25.6	8.6	17
Lentils	21.5	4.5	17
Asparagus	20.8	5.8	15
Figs	18.5		
Corn	17.5	9.5	8
White Beans	27.6	11.6	16
Barley (raw)	17.3		
Prunes (dried, raw)	16.1		
Rolled Oats	15.5	8.5	7
Rye Flour (dark)	14.0		
Coconut	13.6		
Corn Flakes	13.5	7.5	6
Peas	12.0		
Cucumber	11.4	4.4	7
Barley Flour	11.0		
Oat Flour	11.0		
Sweet Potato	10.3	4.3	6
Buckwheat	10.0		
Wholemeal Flour	9.6		
Dates	8.7		
Wholemeal Bread	8.5		
Millet	8.5		
Muesli	7.4		
Baked Beans	7.3		
Oatmeal	7.0		
Rye Flour	7.0		
Apricots	6.7		
Spinach	6.3		
Brown Rice	5.5		
Couscous	5.0		
Butter Beans	5.2		
Broccoli	4.1		

[83] Fiber, Harvard School of Public Health,
http://www.hsph.harvard.edu/nutritionsource/fiber.html
Fiber 101: Soluble fiber vs. insoluble fiber, HealthCastle.com -
http://www.healthcastle.com/fiber-solubleinsoluble.shtml

Leeks	3.9		
Barley	3.8		
Carrots	3.3		
Broccoli	2.9		
Cabbage	2.8		
Brussels Sprouts	2.6	1.2	1.4
Celery	1.7		

The ideal healthy carbohydrate that contains both insoluble and soluble fiber will act to soften blood glucose insulin spike, remove intestinal toxic waste byproducts, and provide an organic source of whole plant food vitamins, minerals, phytonutrients, and antioxidants. Men and women ideally should consume at least 30 grams fiber daily. By choosing plant foods high in fiber, the recommended 55% carbohydrate calorie is less by –6%, converted to 49%, because carbohydrate calories from plant fibers are not digestible. High fiber whole plant foods provide and excellent method to control appetite, blood glucose, and total calorie intake for health.

REFINED CARBOHYDRATES HARMFUL TO HEALTH – Avoid These

Dietary processed form of carbohydrates, with bran, hull, fiber, antioxidants, and phytonutrients removed, compromises health.

For example, simple sugars have been associated with a 2.22-fold increase in breast cancer risk in women who consumed refined carbohydrates, fructose and sucrose. [84] Excess dietary simple sugars have been associated with cancer. [85]

---

[84] Romieu, I., et al. Carbohydrates and the risk of breast cancer among Mexican women. Cancer Epidemiol Biomarkers Prev. 13(8):1283-1289, 2004.

[85] De Stefani, E., et al. Carbohydrates and risk of stomach cancer in Uruguay [letter]. Int J Cancer. 82(4):618-621, 1999; Kaaks, R., et al. Nutrient intake patterns and gastric cancer risk: a case-control study in Belgium. Int J Cancer. 78(4):415-420, 1998; Bostick, R. M., et al. Sugar, meat, and fat intake, and non-dietary risk factors for colon cancer incidence in Iowa women (United States). Cancer Causes Control. 5(1):38-52, 1994; Caderni, G., et al.

Refined carbohydrates have been associated with the prevalence of type 2 diabetes. It has been shown that immediately after eating simple sugars, there is a proportionate loss of vitamin B6, vitamin C, and Magnesium. [86] [87] Excess blood sugar (hyperglycemia) is shown to impair intracellular availability of vitamin C. [88] Whole plant food fiber intake has also been negatively associated with the prevalence of type 2 diabetes. Increasing refined carbohydrates (especially corn syrup) concomitant with less plant food fiber increases type 2 diabetes rates in America. [89]

The major food sources of refined sugars in the USA are soft drinks, breakfast cereals, candy, fruit drinks, and dairy products...[see graph next page]

Dietary sucrose and starch affect dysplastic characteristics in carcinogen-induced aberrant crypt foci in rat colon. Cancer Letters. 114(1-2):39-41, 1997; Luceri, C., et al. Effects of repeated boluses of sucrose on proliferation and on AOM-induced aberrant crypt foci in rat colon. Nutrition & Cancer. 25(2):187-196, 1996.

[86] Seelig, M. Human requirements of magnesium: factors that increase needs. In: First International Symposium on Magnesium Deficiency in Human Pathology. Springer Verlag, Paris. 1971:11.

[87] Leklem, J. E., et al. Acute ingestion of glucose decreases plasma pyridoxal 5'-phosphate and total vitamin B-6 concentration. American Journal of Clinical Nutrition. 51(5):832-836, 1990.

[88] Mann, G. V., et al. The membrane transport of ascorbic acid. Ann NY Acad Sci. 258:243-252, 1975.

[89] Gross, L. S., et al. Increased consumption of refined carbohydrates and the epidemic of type 2 diabetes in the United States: an ecologic assessment. Am J Clin Nutr. 79(5):774-779, 2004.

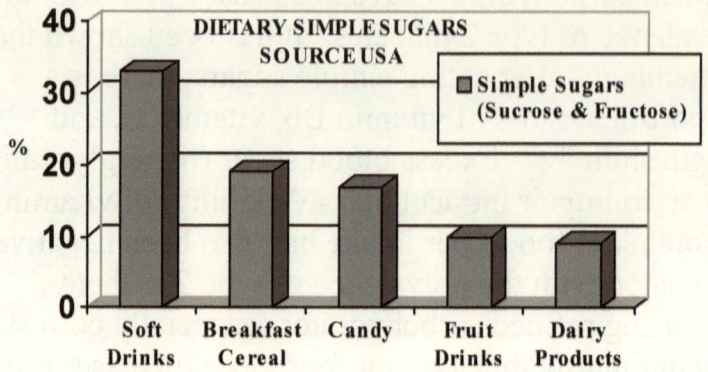

Research shows that diet-induced increased blood sugar is associated with a proportionate increase in diabetes and obesity (next page): [90]

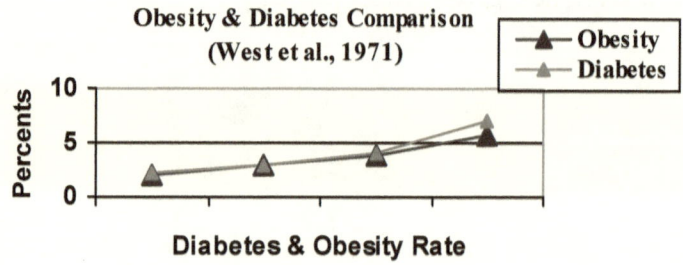

Conversely research reports a remarkable disease-reducing effect in Type I and Type II diabetics simply be changing menu to a plant-based diet (high-fiber, high-carbohydrate, low-fat diet).[91] The recruited patient subjects were normal weight and taking insulin shots to control their blood sugar levels. Notice what the plant food diet did to reduce Type I & II diabetics' blood sugar and total cholesterol levels in only 3-weeks:

[90] West KM, Kalbfleisch JM. "Influence of nutritional factors on prevalence of diabetes." Diabetes 20(1971):99-108.

[91] Anderson JW. "Dietary fiber in nutrition management of diabetes." In: Vahouny GV, Kritchevsky D, eds. Dietary Fiber: Basic andClinical Aspects. New York: Plenum Press, 1986:343-360; Anderson JW, Chen WL, Sieling B. "Hypolipidemic effects of high-carbohydrate, high-fiber diets." Metabolism 29(1980):551-558; Story L, Anderson JW,

Diabetes Type I & II
Response to Plant Food Diet

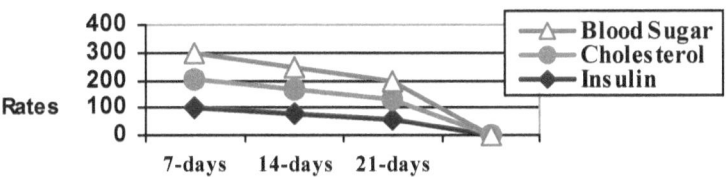

Within 21-days, most Type I diabetic patients (above) were able to lower insulin medication by an average of 40%. The Type II patients in this study were able to discontinue their insulin medication after 3-weeks. The act of medication dose is always done only with the approval of the healthcare Physician. The effect of whole plant food's fiber, antioxidants, and natural complex carbohydrates on restoring normal blood sugar and cholesterol on persons with or without diabetes is quite remarkable.

Chen WL, et al. "Adherence to high-carbohydrate, high-fiber diets: long-term studies of non-obese diabetic men." J Am Diet Assoc. 85(1985):1105-1110; Barnard RJ, Lattimore L, Holly RG, et al. "Response of non-insulin-dependent diabetic patients to an intensive program of diet and exercise." Diabetes Care 5(1982):370-374.

Any food or drink containing sugars (or easily complex carbohydrate starch, etc.) will cause blood glucose levels to increase. Increasing blood sugar causes the pancreas to release insulin to provide a carrier for sweeping blood sugars into cells. Insulin causes the insulin-sensitive tissues in muscle cells or fat cells to absorb glucose in order to lower blood glucose. As the blood glucose levels decrease, less insulin is required. The problem is that in time and with repeated exposure to diet-induced high blood sugar, a person may become insulin-resistant and normal levels of insulin will fail to control blood glucose. When insulin resistance occurs and blood glucose is not controlled effectively, impaired fasting glucose or impaired glucose tolerance concentrations increase the risk of Diabetes type II. Repeated exposures to elevated insulin may also cause additional health disorders.

Overweight and obesity are associated with insulin resistance. Research stated, "When hyperglycemia develops after a meal, when pancreatic beta-cells are unable to produce sufficient insulin to maintain normal blood sugar levels (euglycemia) in the face of insulin resistance. The inability of the beta-cells to produce sufficient insulin in a condition of hyperglycemia is what characterizes the transition from insulin resistance to Type 2 diabetes mellitus." [92] Nancy Appleton, PhD, author, aptly listed 76-ways dietary sugar can inhibit health. [93]

---

[92] McGarry J (2002). "Banting lecture 2001: dysregulation of fatty acid metabolism in the etiology of type 2 diabetes". Diabetes 51 (1): 7–18.
[93] Appleton N. Lick the Sugar Habit (1996) Avery, 2nd Ed. 272 pp.

Common whole plant foods fruits and vegetables contain 7-30% total carbohydrate but only 0.5-15% as simple sugar. However, when a whole plant food fruit or vegetable is processed, it can be converted from 15% sugar to a whooping 100% juice, consisting of granulated sugar sweetener, resulting in the original 15% simple sugar content to become 90% of the food's total calories. Such processed foods provoke a high blood sugar high insulin response including a negative effect on health.

PRACTICAL APPLICATIONS CARBOHYDRATES - What do I do?

➤ Consume only whole plant food fruit and vegetables.
➤ Do not consume processed fruit juices and refined simple sugars from diet.
➤ Do not consume soft drinks, candy, refined high sugar breakfast cereals, dairy, and fruit juices from diet. Read the labels….
➤ Consume at least 30-35 grams fiber daily.
➤ Consume approximately 1000 carbohydrate calories daily from whole plant foods. Work rate or exercise calorie expense justifies increasing dose at 100 calories per mile or 100 calories per 15 minutes aerobic work rate.
➤ Do not consume fiber-empty calories from a source that is more 15% calories refined or simple sugars.
➤ The carbohydrate dietary goal is to supply energy upon demand and maintain normal blood glucose levels. Whole plant foods meet this goal; processed foods may not meet this goal.

CHAPTER VI - FOODS FOR HEALTH

UN-processed, UN-refined whole plant foods provide a rich assortment of bran-hull fibers, antioxidants, and phytonutrients that enhance health and prevent diseases. Consuming whole plant foods recommended from vegetable families Beets, Cabbage, Gourd, Nightshade, Onion, & Parsley are reported to generate a number of health functions as follows:

BEET FAMILY vegetables such as beetroot, silver beets, spinach, and sugar beets have been associated with prevention of several forms of cancers of the colon, liver, lung, prostate, skin, stomach, and uterus. Beets eradicate the Hepatitis C virus. Beetroot vegetables lower elevated total serum cholesterol. Beetroot vegetables may improve liver function by stimulating the regeneration of liver tissue and by stimulating the dietary fat metabolism. [1-8]

CABBAGE FAMILY vegetables such as broccoli, brussel sprouts, cabbage, cauliflower, chinese broccoli, choy sum, daikon, kale, kohlrabi, mustard greens, radish, rutabaga, turnips have been associated with prevention of colon, lung, prostate, bladder, breast, & cervical cancer. [9-13]

GOURD FAMILY vegetables such as cucumber, pumpkin, summer squash, winter squash, & zucchini high-carotenoid content have been associated with reduced risk of prostate cancer and diabetes. [14-16]

PARSLEY FAMILY vegetables such as carrots, celery, fennel, parsnip, and parsley are associated with reducing the risks of colon, mouth, and lung cancers, reducing risk of heart disease by lowering total cholesterol, reducing the risk of diabetes, reducing the prevalence asthma, reducing the risk of psoriasis, and reducing risk of Candida albicans. [17-25]

NIGHTSHADE FAMILY vegetables such as eggplant, potato, tomato, & chilli peppers have been associated with reducing total cholesterol and cardiovascular heart disease, preventing of several forms of colon, esophageal, lung, mouth, pancreatic, prostate, and stomach cancers, reducing PSA levels, lowering total cholesterol, decreasing elevated blood pressure, reducing the risk of asthma and emphysema, reducing the risk of psoriasis and the risk of thrombotic (blood clotting) events. [26-44]

ONION FAMILY vegetables chives garlic, leeks, and onions have been associated with reduced rate of aging, improved circulation, reduced elevated blood pressure, reduced risk of cancers, reduce risk pf stroke, and enhanced immune system resistance against harmful microbes. [45-62]

Cited References for vegetable whole plant foods above (1-62):

1. Kapadia, G. J., et al. Chemoprevention of lung and skin cancer by Beta vulgaris (beet) root extract. Cancer Lett. 100(1-2):211-214, 1996.
2. Morant, R., et al. Why do cancer patients use alternative medicine? Schweiz Med Wochenschr. 121(27-28):1029-1034, 1991.

3. Obrist, R., et al. The use of paramedical treatment methods by cancer patients. An inquiry on 101 ambulatory patients. Dtsch Med Wochenschr. 111(8):283-287, 1986.
4. Seeger, P. G. Arzliche Forschung. 21:68-78, 1967.
5. Tyihak, E. Naturwissenschaften. 51:315-316, 1964; & Revista Brasilica de Biologia. 40:519-244, 1980.
6. Konlee, M. Case report: Beets helped reduce Hepatitis (HCV viral load). Journal of Immunity. 4(4), 2006.
7. Bobek, P., et al. The effect of red beet (Beta vulgaris var. rubra) fiber on alimentary hypercholesterolemia and chemically induced colon carcinogenesis in rats. Nahrung. 44(3):184-187, 2000.
8. Agarwal, M., et al. Hepatoprotective activity of Beta vulgaris against CCl(4)-induced hepatic injury in rats. Fitoterapia. 77(2):91-93, 2006.
9. Hecht, S. S. Inhibition of carcinogenesis by isothiocyanates. Drug Metab Rev. 32(3-4):395-411, 2000.
10. Talalay, P., et al. Phytochemicals from cruciferous plants protect against cancer by modulating carcinogen metabolism. Journal of Nutrition. 131(11 Supplement):3027S-3033S, 2001.
11. Verhoeven, D. T., et al. Epidemiological studies on brassica vegetables and cancer risk. Cancer Epidemiology, Biomarkers and Prevention. 5(9):733-748, 1996

12. Kassie, F., et al. Chemoprevention of 2-amino-3-methylimidazo[4,5-f]quinoline (IQ)-induced colonic and hepatic preneoplastic lesions in the F344 rat by cruciferous vegetables administered simultaneously with the carcinogen. Carcinogenesis. 24(2):255-261, 2003.

13. Walters, D. G., et al. Cruciferous vegetable consumption alters the metabolism of the dietary carcinogen 2-amino-1-methyl-6-phenylimidazo[4,5-b]pyridine (PhIP) in humans. Carcinogenesis. 2004.

14. Binns, C. W., et al. The relationship between dietary carotenoids and prostate cancer risk in Southeast Chinese men. Asia Pac J Clin Nutr. 13(Supplement):S117, 2004.

15. Jian, L., et al. Do dietary lycopene and other carotenoids protect against prostate cancer? Int J Cancer. 2004.

16. Suzuki, K., et al. Relationship between serum carotenoids and hyperglycemia: a population-based cross-sectional study. J Epidemiol. 12(5):357-366, 2002.

17. Slattery, M., et al. Carotenoids and colon cancer. American Journal of Clinical Nutrition. 71(2):575-582, 2000.

18. van Breda, S. G., et al. Vegetables affect the expression of genes involved in carcinogenic and anticarcinogenic processes in the lungs of female C57BL/6 mice. Journal of Nutrition. 135(11):2546-2552, 2005.

19. Fioretti, F., et al. Risk factors for oral and pharyngeal cancer in never smokers. Oral Oncol. 35(4):375-378, 1999.

20. Nicolle, C., et al. Effect of carrot intake on cholesterol metabolism and on antioxidant status in cholesterol-fed rat. Eur J Nutr. 42(5):254-261, 2003.
21. Robertson, J., et al. The effect of raw carrot on serum lipids and colon function. American Journal of Clinical Nutrition. 32(9):1889-1892, 1978.
22. Suzuki, K., et al. Relationship between serum carotenoids and hyperglycemia: a population-based cross-sectional study. J Epidemiol. 12(5):357-366, 2002.
23. Romieu, I., et al. Fruit and vegetable intakes and asthma in the E3N study. Thorax. 61(3):209-215, 2006.
24. Naldi, L., et al. Dietary factors and the risk of psoriasis. Results of an Italian case-control study. British Journal of Dermatology. 134(1):101-106, 1996.
25. Amin, M., et al. Carrot phytoalexin alters the membrane permeability of Candida albicans and multilamellar liposomes. Journal of General Microbiology. 134(Pt 1):241-246, 1988.
26. Mitschek, G. H. Effect of Solanum melongena on experimental atheromatosis. VI. Enzyme histochemical, physiopathological and chemical studies on cholesterol-induced atheromatosis in rabbits. Conclusions. Experimentelle Pathelogie. 10(3-4):167-179, 1975.
27. Franceschi, S., et al. Tomatoes and risk of digestive-tract cancer. Int J Cancer. 59(2):181-184, 1994.
28. Sengupta, A., et al. Tomato and garlic can modulate azoxymethane-induced colon carcinogenesis in rats. Eur J Cancer Prev. 12(3):195-200, 2003.

29. Binns, C. W., et al. The relationship between dietary carotenoids and prostate cancer risk in Southeast Chinese men. Asia Pac J Clin Nutr. 13(Supplement):S117, 2004.
30. Campbell, J. K., et al. Tomato phytochemicals and prostate cancer risk. Journal of Nutrition. 134(12):3486S-3492S, 2004.
31. Durak, I., et al. Tomato juice inhibits adenosine deaminase activity in human prostate tissue from patient with prostate cancer. Nutrition Research. 23(9):1183-1188, 2003.
32. Ellinger, S., et al. Tomatoes, tomato products and lycopene in the prevention and treatment of prostate cancer: do we have the evidence from intervention studies? Curr Opin Clin Nutr Metab Care. 9(6):722-727, 2006.
33. Jian, L., et al. Do dietary lycopene and other carotenoids protect against prostate cancer? Int J Cancer. 2004.
34. Edinger, M. S., et al. Effect of the consumption of tomato paste on plasma prostate-specific antigen levels in patients with benign prostate hyperplasia. Braz J Med Biol Res. 39(8):1115-1119, 2006.
35. Hsu, Y. M., et al. Characterizing the lipid-lowering effects and antioxidant mechanisms of tomato paste. Biosci Biotechnol Biochem. 2008.
36. Romieu, I., et al. Fruit and vegetable intakes and asthma in the E3N study. Thorax. 61(3):209-215, 2006.
37. Kasagi, S., et al. Tomato juice prevents from developing emphysema induced by chronic exposure to tobacco smoke in senescence-accelerated mouse P1 strain. Am J Physiol Lung Cell Mol Physiol. 2005.

38. Englehard, Y. N., et al. Natural antioxidants from tomato extract reduce blood pressure in patients with grade-1 hypertension: a double-blind, placebo-controlled pilot study. American Heart Journal. 151(1):100, 2006.

39. Naldi, L., et al. Dietary factors and the risk of psoriasis. British Journal of Dermatology.134(1):101-106, 1996.

40. O'Kennedy, N., et al. Effects of tomato extract on platelet function: a double-blinded crossover study in healthy humans. American Journal of Clinical Nutrition. 84(3):561-569, 2006.

41. Moriguchi, T., et al. Anti-ageing effect of aged garlic in the inbred brain atrophy mouse model. Clin Exp Pharmacol Physiol. 24(3-4):235-242, 1997.

42. Svendsen, L., et al. Testing garlic for possible anti-ageing effects on long term growth characteristics, morphology and macromolecular synthesis of human fibroblasts in culture. Journal of Ethnopharmacology. 43(2):125-133, 1994.

43. Khosh, F. Natural approach to hypertension. Alternative Medicine Review. 6(6), 2001.

44. Kiesewetter, H., et al. Effect of garlic on thrombocyte aggregation, microcirculation, and other risk factors. Int J Clin Pharmacol Ther Toxicol. 29(4):151-155, 1991.

45. Korotkov, V. M. The action of garlic juice on blood pressure. Vrachebnoe Deioebnoe. 6:123, 1966.

46. Leoper, M., et al. Hypotensive effect of tincture of garlic. Prog Med. 36:391-392, 1921.

47. McMahon, F. G., et al. Can garlic lower blood pressure? A pilot study. Pharmacotherapy. 13(4):406-407, 1993.

48. Hsing, A. W., et al. Allium vegetables and risk of prostate cancer: a population-based study. J Natl Cancer Inst. 94(21):1648-1651, 2002.
49. Kim, J. M., et al. Dietary S-allyl-l-cysteine reduces mortality with decreased incidence of stroke and behavioral changes in stroke-prone spontaneously hypertensive rats. Biosci Biotechnol Biochem. 70(8):1969-1971, 2006.
50. Siegel, G., et al. [Pleiotropic effects of garlic.] Wien Med Wochenschr. 149(8-10):217-224, 1999.
51. Yamada, N., et al. Prophylactic effects of ajoene on cerebral injury in stroke-prone spontaneously hypertensive rats (SHRSP). Biol Pharm Bull. 29(4):619-622, 2006.
52. Das, S. Garlic - a natural source of cancer preventive compounds. Asian Pac J Cancer Prev. 3(4):305-311, 2002.
53. Knowles, L. M., et al. Possible mechanism by which allyl sulfides suppress neoplastic cell proliferation. Journal of Nutrition. 131:1061S-1066S, 2001.
54. Kuttan, R., et al. Tumour reducing and anticarcinogenic activity of selected spices. Cancer Letters. 51:85-89, 1990.
55. Lau, B., et al. Allium sativum and cancer prevention. Nutr Res. 10:937-948, 1990.
56. Lea, M. A., et al. International Journal of Oncology. 11(1):181-185, 1997.
57. Milner, J. A. Mechanisms by which garlic and allyl sulfur compounds suppress carcinogen bioactivation. Garlic and carcinogenesis. Adv Exp Med Biol. 492:69-81, 2001.

58. Milner, J. A. A historical perspective on garlic and cancer. Journal of Nutrition. 131(3 Supplement):1027S-1031S, 2001.
59. Nagini, S. Cancer chemoprevention by garlic and its organosulfur compounds-panacea or promise? Anticancer Agents Med Chem. 8(3):313-321, 2008.
60. Oommen, S., et al. Allicin (from garlic) induces caspase-mediated apoptosis in cancer cells. Eur J Pharmacol. 485(1-3):97-103, 2004.
61. Shukla, Y., et al. Cancer chemoprevention with garlic and its constituents. Cancer Letters. 2006.
62. Harris, J. C., et al. Antimicrobial properties of Allium sativum (garlic). Appl Microbiol Biotechnol. 57(3):282-286, 2001.

Dr. Joel Fuhrman's ANDI Scoring System [94]

The Fuhrman ANDI (Aggregate Nutrient Density Index) ranks foods based on the ratio of nutrients to calories. Nutrient Density is a critical concept in devising and recommending dietary and nutritional advice to patients and to the public. Not merely vitamins and minerals, but adequate consumption of phytochemicals are essential for proper functioning of the immune system and to enable our body's detoxification and cellular repair mechanisms that protect us from chronic diseases. Nutritional science in the last twenty years has demonstrated that colorful plant foods contain a huge assortment of protective compounds, most of which still remain unnamed.

---

[94] Dr. Fuhrman's nutrient density food rankings, scoring system, and point determinations of foods and dietary application to individual medical needs is patented. The patent is held by Dr. Fuhrman and Kevin Leville of Eat Right America.

Only by eating an assortment of nutrient-rich natural foods can we access these protective compounds and prevent the common diseases that afflict Americans. Our modern, low-nutrient eating style has led to an overweight population, the majority of whom develop diseases of nutritional ignorance, causing our medical costs to spiral out of control. To guide people toward the most nutrient dense foods, Dr. Joel Fuhrman developed a remarkable scoring system called ANDI (Aggregate Nutrient Density Index), which ranks foods based on their ratio of nutrients to calories.

Because phytochemicals are largely unnamed and unmeasured, these rankings underestimate the healthful properties of colorful natural plant foods compared to processed foods and animal products. One thing we do know is that the foods that contain the highest amount of known nutrients are the same foods that contain the most unknown nutrients too. So even though these rankings may not consider the phytochemical number sufficiently, they are still a reasonable measurement of their content. Keep in mind that nutrient density scoring is not the only factor that determines good health. For example, if we only ate foods with a high nutrient density score our diet would be too low in fat.
So we have to pick some foods with lower nutrient density scores (but preferably the healthier ones) to include in our high nutrient diet. Additionally, if a slim or highly physically active individual ate only the highest nutrient foods they would become so full from all of the fiber and nutrients that would keep them from meeting their caloric needs and they would eventually become too thin.

This of course gives you a hint at the secret to permanent weight control – to eat the greatest quantity of the foods with the highest ANDI scores, and lesser amounts of foods with lower ANDI scores. For further information, read chapter 3 in EAT FOR HEALTH, in which Dr. Fuhrman discusses nutrient density and the importance of phytochemicals in detail.

To determine the scores above almost all vitamins and minerals were considered and added in. Nutrient Data from Nutritionist Pro software for an equal caloric amount of each food item was obtained. We included the following nutrients in the evaluation: Calcium, Carotenoids: Beta Carotene, Alpha Carotene, Lutein & Zeaxanthin, Lycopene, Fiber, Folate, Glucosinolates, Iron, Magnesium, Niacin, Selenium, Vitamin B1 (Thiamin) Vitamin B2 (Riboflavin), Vitamin B6, Vitamin B12, Vitamin C, Vitamin E, Zinc, plus ORAC score X 2 (Oxygen Radical Absorbance Capacity is a method of measuring the antioxidant or radical scavenging capacity of foods). Nutrient quantities, which are normally in many different measurements (mg, mcg, IU) were converted to a percentage of their RDI so that a common value could be considered for each nutrient. Since there is currently no RDI for Carotenoids, Glucosinolates, or ORAC score, goals were established based on available research and current understanding of the benefits of these factors. (limited references below). The % RDI or Goal for each nutrient, which the USDA publishes a value for, was added together to give a total. All nutrients were weighted equally with a factor of one except for the foods ORAC score. The ORAC score was given a factor 2 (as if it were two nutrients) due to the importance of antioxidant phytonutrients so that a contribution from unnamed and unscored anti-oxidant phytochemicals were represented in the scoring. The sum of the food's total nutrient value was then multiplied by a fraction to make the highest number equal 1000 so that all foods could be considered on a numerical scale of 1 to 1000.

The green column (left) shows preferred nutrient-dense whole plant foods, the middle column shows foods with less nutrient density, and the outside (right) column shows foods with the least nutrient density. Dr. Fuhrman's ANDI Scoring System rationale is well supported and may be used to rotate whole healthy plant foods for health-sustaining effects:

Dr. Fuhrman ANDI Scoring System: Sample Scores [95]

Kale	1000	Cantaloupe	100	Skim Milk	36
Collards	1000	Kidney Beans	100	Walnuts	34
Bok Choy	824	Sweet Potato	83	Grapes	31
Spinach	739	Black Beans	83	White Potato	31
Broccoli Rabe	715	Sunflower Seeds	78	Banana	30
Chinese/Napa Cabbage	704	Apple	76	Cashews	27
Brussel Sprouts	672	Peach	73	Chicken Breast	27
Swiss Chard	670	Green Peas	70	Eggs	27
Arugula	559	Cherries	68	Peanut Butter	26
Cabbage	481	Flax Seeds	65	Whole Wheat Bread	25
Romaine Lettuce	389	Pineapple	64	Feta Cheese	21
Broccoli	376	Chick Peas	57	Whole Milk	20
Carrot Juice	344	Oatmeal	53	Ground Beef	20
Cauliflower	295	Pumpkin Seeds	52	White Pasta	18
Green Peppers	258	Mango	51	White Bread	18
Artichoke	244	Cucumber	50	Apple Juice	16
Carrots	240	Soybeans	48	Swiss Cheese	15
Asparagus	234	Pistachio Nuts	48	Low Fat Yogurt	14
Strawberries	212	Corn	44	Potato Chips	11
Pomegranate Juice	193	Brown Rice	41	American Cheese	10
Tomato	164	Salmon	39	Vanilla Ice Cream	9
Blueberries	130	Almonds	38	French Fries	7
Iceberg Lettuce	110	Shrimp	38	Olive Oil	2
Orange	109	Avocado	37	Cola	1
Lentils	100	Tofu	37		

Joel Fuhrman, M.D.

References for Dr. Fuhrman ANDI Scoring System:

- Nutritionist Pro [Nutrition Analysis Software] Versions 2.5, 3.1. Stafford TX . Axxya Systems. 2005,2006.
- Higdon, Jane. Isothiocyanates. The Linus Pauling Institute. Micronutrient Research Center. 9/20/2005. http://oregonstate.edu/infocenter/phytochemicals/isothio.
- Wu, Xianli; Beecher, Gary; Holden, Joanne; Haytowitz, David; Gebhardt, Susan; Prior Ronald. 2004; Lipophilic and Hydrophilic Antioxidant Capacities of Common Foods in the United States. Journal of Agricultural and Food Chemistry. 52. 4026-4037.
- Dietary Reference Intakes for Vitamin C, Vitamin E, Selenium, and Caroteinoids, 2000. Food and Nutrition Board. Institute of Medicine. National Academy Press. Washington D.C. pp. 343-344.
- Dietary Reference Intakes for Energy, Carbohydrate, Fiber, Fat, Fatty Acids, Cholesterol, Protein, and Amino Acids. 2002. Food and Nutrition Board. Institute of Medicine. National Academy Press. Washington D.C. p. 423.
- Mc Bride, Judy. 1999. Can Foods Forestall Aging? Agricultural Research. 47(2): 15-17.
- Wu, Xianli; Beecher, Gary; Holden, Joanne; Haytowitz, David; Gebhardt, Susan; Prior, Ronald. 2004. Lipophilic and Hydrophilic Antioxidant Capacities of Common Foods in the United States.
Journal of Agricultural and Food Chemistry. 52. 4026-4037.

➤ Prior, Ronald. Hoang, Ha. Gu, Liwei. Bacchiocca, Mara. Howard, Luke. Hanpsch-Woodill, Maureen. Huang, Dejuan. Ou, Boxin, Jacob, Robert. 2003. Assays for Hydrophilic and Lipophilic Antioxidant Capacity of Plasma and Other Biological and Food Samples. Journal of Agricultural and Food Chemistry. 51. 3273-3279.

➤ Dietary Reference Intakes for Vitamin C, Vitamin E, Selenium and Caroteinoids. 2000. Food and Nutrition Board. Institiute of Medicine. National Academy Press. Washington D.C. pp. 343-344. Prior, RL. 1999. Can Foods Forestall Aging? Agricultural Research. 47(2): 15-17.

PRACTICAL APPLICATIONS WHOLE PLANT FOODS - What do I do?

How much and what whole plant foods should supply half of our calories (50-55% as carbohydrates)? This is an important question. Consuming foods that provide a minimum of 30-35 grams fiber per day and a minimum of 5000 ORAC units, and the highest phytonutrient content are both health enhancing and disease-preventive. The table following ranks foods based on fiber, antioxidant potency (Oxygen Radical Absorbance Capacity - ORAC), and the Fuhrman ANDI Scores phytonutrient values:

FOOD (Rank high to lowest)	FIBER % PER 100 GRAMS	FOOD (Rank high to lowest)	ANTIOXIDANT POTENCY (ORAC) PER 100 GRAMS	FOOD (Rank high to lowest)	Fuhrman ANDI Scoring System88
Wheat Bran	46.6	Prunes	5,770	Kale	1000
Flax Seeds	32.0	Pomegranates	3,307	Collards	1000
Oat Bran	30.3	Raisins	2,830	Bok Choy	824
White Beans	27.6	Blueberries	2,400	Spinach	739
Pinto Beans	27.2	Blackberries	2,036	Broccoli Rabe	715

Food	Value	Food	Value	Food	Value
Kale	25.9	Garlic	1,939	Chinese/Napa Cabbage	704
Lima Beans	25.6	Kale	1,770	Brussel Sprouts	672
Lentils	21.5	Cranberries	1,750	Swiss Chard	670
Asparagus	20.8	Strawberries	1,540	Arugula	559
Figs	18.5	Spinach	1,260	Cabbage	481
Corn	17.5	Raspberries	1,220	Romaine Lettuce	389
White Beans	27.6	Yellow Squash	1,150	Broccoli	376
Barley (raw)	17.3	Brussels Sprouts	980	Carrots	344
Prunes	16.1	Plums	949	Cauliflower	295
Rolled Oats	15.5	Alfalfa Sprouts	930	Green Peppers	258
Coconut	13.6	Steamed Spinach	909	Artichoke	244
Corn Flakes	13.5	Broccoli	890	Asparagus	234
Peas	12.0	Beets	840	Strawberries	212
Cucumber	11.4	Avocado	782	Pomegranate Juice	193
Sweet Potato	10.3	Oranges	750	Tomato	164
Buckwheat	10.0	Grapes, Red	739	Blueberries	130
Dates	8.7	Red Bell Pepper	710	Iceberg Lettuce	110
Wholemeal Bread	8.5	Cherries	670	Orange	109
Millet	8.5	Kiwi Fruit	610	Lentils, Cantaloupe, Kidney Beans	100
Muesli	7.4	Beans, Baked	503	Sweet Potato	83
Baked Beans	7.3	Grapefruit, Pink	495	Black Beans	83
Oatmeal	7.0	Grapes, White	460	Sweet Potato	83
Rye Flour	7.0	Beans, Kidney	460	Sunflower Seeds	78
Apricots	6.7	Onion	450	Apple	76
Spinach	6.3	Corn	400	Peach	73
Brown Rice	5.5	Eggplant	390	Green Peas	70
Couscous	5.0	Cauliflower	385	Cherries	68
Butter Beans	5.2	Peas, Frozen	375	Flax Seeds	65
Broccoli	4.1	Potato	300	Pineapple	64
Leeks	3.9	Sweet Potato	295	Chick Peas	57
Barley	3.8	Cabbage	295	Oatmeal	53
Carrots	3.3	Leaf Lettuce	265	Pumpkin Seeds	52
Broccoli	2.9	Cantaloupe	250	Mango	51
Cabbage	2.8	Banana	210	Cucumber	50
Brussels Sprouts	2.6	Apple	207	Soybeans	48
Celery	1.7	Tofu, Carrots, String Beans, & Tomato	195-205	Pistachio Nuts	48

DR BILL'S - TOP 15 FOODS: Based on the combined ratings for food's fiber content, food's ORAC antioxidant content, and food's nutrient ANDI score, the following foods are my favorites to be included in the menu on a regular basis:

1. Kale
2. Prunes
3. Pomegranates
4. Berries
5. Beans
6. Asparagus
7. Spinach
8. Lentils
9. Rolled Oats/Oat Bran
10. Peppers
11. Beets
12. Brussel Sprouts
13. Broccoli
14. Cauliflower
15. Carrots

.

CHAPTER VII FOOD SYNERGY

Why should we consume plant foods and avoid animal source foods? The answer is "Synergy Effects," defined as the physical inter-action between multiple substances so that their combined effect is greater than the sum of less than the separated parts. "Synergy Effect" from harmful substances simultaneously compounds the degree of harm as substance exposure increases. One toxic substance might be tolerated or neutralized by our immune system, but as toxins increase, the risk to compromised health increases exponentially with each harmful substance added. Conversely, required nutrients magnify the healthful effects of the others. The sum of all the nutrients far exceeds individual the effects of one. "Synergy Effects" based on what we eat suggest that multiple substances multiply either good healthful effects or bad toxic unhealthful effects.

SYNERGY TOXIC SUBSTANCE EFFECT

The more toxic substances exposed to, the more likely a toxic effect. One substance may be tolerated and resolved by the immune system, but as toxic substances increase, the harmful effects are multiplied, potentially compromising health or ending life. An example is: "Immature male rats were fed a purified, low-fiber diet to which were added these substances individually or in combination:

2% sodium cyclamate
2% FD&C Red No. 2
4% polyoxyethylene (20) sorbitan monostearate

Whereas supplements of any one of these three food additives indicated above had little if any deleterious effect, combined supplements of sodium cyclamate and FDK Red No. 2 resulted in a marked retardation in weight increment, an unthrifty appearance of the fur, alopecia and extensive diarrhea with watery and mushy stools. Concurrent administration of all three-food additives resulted in a further retardation in weight increment and death of all test animals within an experimental period of 14 days. " [96] [97]

While Professor Campbell's research demonstrated that the whole plant food lifestyle is associated with health, it is noted that only a few percentage point deviations increase risk of disease. [98] When calorie intake from animal-source foods exceeded 5% of the total, pre-cancer foci cells occur. With each additional +1% animal-source calories, foci cells increased, identifying culprit. Less calories from animal-source foods is better than more.

Synergy Health Effect Plant Foods
Similarly, a favorable health effect occurs from only eating plant foods. As bad as the harmful effect is from eating toxic substances, so is the good effect magnified by eating healthful substances from a variety of whole plant foods.

---

[96] Ershoff BH. Synergistic Toxicity of Food Additives in Rats Fed a Diet Low in Dietary Fiber. Journal of Food Science Vol. 41: 4. 949-951 1976.
[97] "The deleterious effects obtained on the latter diet could be largely counteracted by the concurrent administration of various dietary fiber-containing materials. Blond psyllium seed powder was particularly potent in this regard. The protective factor or factors therein was distinct from any of the known nutrients and from cellulose per se." Fiber is contained only in plant foods. Interesting to the author that plant fibers reduce the harmful effect of manmade food additives that otherwise unrestricted result in death.
[98] Campbell TC. Campbell TM. *The China Study*. Benbella Books. Dallas, Texas; pp 52-53.

Liu stated: "The combination of orange, apple, grape, and blueberry displayed a synergistic effect in antioxidant activity The dose–response curve of antioxidant activity was shifted to the left after the combination of 4 fruits. The median effective dose (EC_{50}) of each fruit after combination was 5 times lower than the EC_{50} of each fruit alone, suggesting synergistic effects after the combination of the 4 fruits. Therefore, consumers should obtain their phytochemicals from a wide variety of fruits, vegetables, and whole grains for optimal health benefits."

A researcher (figure 7) demonstrated that a variety of whole plant foods increases the relative antioxidant effects significantly compared to a single plant food.

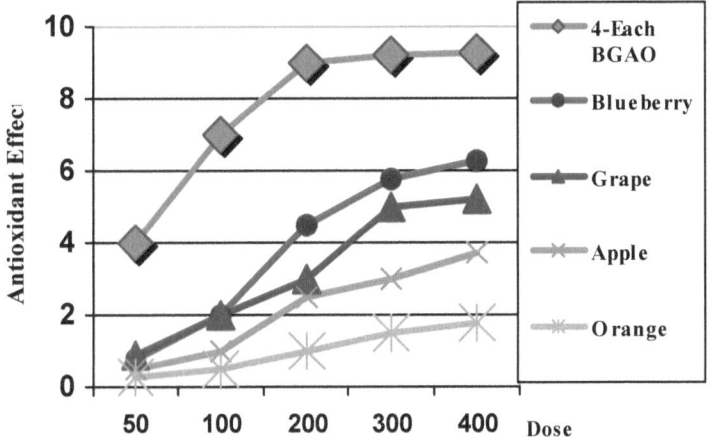

Figure 7. Synergy Effect: Compare the dose response antioxidant activity of a 4-way combination (■), blueberry (●), grape (▼), apple (✕), and orange (✳). [99]
The 4-way dose combination of the whole produces 200-800 % greater antioxidant effect than a single fruit.

[99] Liu RH. Health benefits of fruit and vegetables are from additive and synergistic combinations of phytochemicals. Am J Clin Nutr. 2003 Sep;78(3 Suppl):517S-520S.

Liu added: "In 2003 Temple and Gladwin reviewed > 200 cohort and case-control studies that provided risk ratios concerning intake of fruits and vegetables and risk of cancer. They concluded that cancer prevention is best achieved by consumption of a wide variety of fruits and vegetables, although one group of fruits and vegetables may dominate for a particular cancer. [100] To improve their nutrition and health, consumers should be obtaining antioxidants from their diet and not from expensive dietary supplements, which do not contain the balanced combination of phytochemicals found in fruits and vegetables and other whole foods.

More importantly, obtaining antioxidants from dietary intake by consuming a wide variety of foods is unlikely to result in consumption of toxic quantities, because foods originating from plants contain many diverse types of phytochemicals in various quantities. Fruits and vegetables eaten in the recommended amounts (5-10 servings of fruits and vegetables per day) are safe. Furthermore, health benefits from the consumption of fruits and vegetables extend beyond lowering the risk of developing cancers and CVD: benefits also include preventive effects on other chronic diseases such as cataracts, age-related macular degeneration, central neurodegenerative diseases, and diabetes." [101]

---

[100] Temple, N. J. & Gladwin, K. K. (2003) Fruits, vegetables, and the prevention of cancer: research challenges. Nutrition 19:467-470.
[101] Liu RH. Health benefits of fruit and vegetables are from additive and synergistic combinations of phytochemicals. Am J Clin Nutr. 2003 Sep;78(3 Suppl):517S-520S.

Liu concluded: "The additive and synergistic effects of phytochemicals in fruits and vegetables are responsible for their potent antioxidant and anticancer activities. The benefit of a diet rich in fruits, vegetables, and whole grains is attributed to the complex mixture of phytochemicals present in these and other whole foods. This is why a single antioxidant cannot effectively replace the combination of natural phytochemicals in fruits and vegetables to achieve the same health benefits. The evidence suggests that antioxidants are best acquired through whole food consumption, not from expensive dietary supplements. Further research on the health benefits of phytochemicals in whole foods is warranted." [102]

Synergy Whole Food Effects – Health or Compromised Health

The evidence of whole foods synergy imposed potency effect on human health deserves consideration. A recurrent theme appears, plant foods are associated with a proportionate decreased risk of disease, while consuming animal source foods has been associated with an increased risk of disease:

The synergy effect from a whole food is greater than any part. The action of the food matrix on human biological systems is greater than or different from the corresponding actions of the individual food components.

Research summarizes that to attain ideal health benefits, the combination of food components needs to address their interactions within the food and with the human system:

---

[102] Ibid.

➤ Food components must survive digestion to arrive in such a way that the mutual effects of the different components can be realized after eating. (Jacobs DR Jr, Gross MD, Tapsell LC. Food synergy: an operational concept for understanding nutrition. Am J Clin Nutr. 2009) May;89(5):1543S-1548S. Epub 2009 Mar 11. Review.)

➤ Epidemiological studies have shown that consumption of fruits and vegetables is associated with reduced risk of chronic disease. Increased consumption of plant foods with their phytochemical content has been proposed to prevent chronic diseases related to oxidative stress in humans. Researchers measured phenolic content in 10 common vegetables selected on the basis of consumption per person in the USA. The highest total *Phenolic* content from highest to lowest in the following whole plant foods: broccoli spinach, yellow onion, red pepper, carrot, cabbage, potato, lettuce, celery, and cucumber. (Chu, Y.-F., Sun, J., Wu, X. & Liu, R. H. (2002) Antioxidant and antiproliferative activities of vegetables. J. Agric. Food Chem. 50: 6910–6916.)

➤ Researchers measured total *Antioxidant* content from highest to lowest in the following whole plant foods: red pepper, broccoli, carrot, spinach, cabbage, yellow onion, celery, potato, lettuce, and cucumber. (Chu, Y.-F., Sun, J., Wu, X. & Liu, R. H. (2002) Antioxidant and antiproliferative activities of vegetables. J. Agric. Food Chem. 50: 6910–6916.)

➢ Researchers measured the *Antiproliferative* effects of whole plant foods in human liver cancer cells. Spinach showed the highest inhibitory antiproliferative effect, followed by cabbage, red pepper, onion, and broccoli. On the basis of these results, the bioactivity index (BI) for dietary cancer prevention is proposed to provide a simple reference for consumers to choose vegetables in accordance with their beneficial activities. (Chu, Y.-F., Sun, J., Wu, X. & Liu, R. H. (2002) Antioxidant and antiproliferative activities of vegetables. J. Agric. Food Chem. 50: 6910–6916.)

➢ Phytochemicals phenolic compound in whole the following whole plant foods are bioactive compounds for the health benefits. Researchers measured total phenolics in common fruits. The following whole plant foods from highest-to-lowest *Phenolic* content were cranberry, apple, red grape, strawberry, pineapple, banana, peach, lemon, orange, pear, and grapefruit. (Sun, J., Chu, Y.-F., Wu, X. & Liu, R. H. (2002) Antioxidant and antiproliferative activities of fruits. J. Agric. Food Chem. 50: 7449–7454.)

➢ Total *Antioxidant* activity was measured showing that Cranberry had the highest total antioxidant activity followed by apple, red grape, strawberry, peach, lemon, pear, banana, orange, grapefruit, and pineapple. (Sun, J., Chu, Y.-F., Wu, X. & Liu, R. H. (2002) Antioxidant and antiproliferative activities of fruits. J. Agric. Food Chem. 50: 7449–7454.)

➤ The following whole plant foods produced *Antiproliferation* effects against human liver-cancer cells, from highest to lowest cranberry, lemon, apple, strawberry, red grape, banana, grapefruit, and peach. (Sun, J., Chu, Y.-F., Wu, X. & Liu, R. H. (2002) Antioxidant and antiproliferative activities of fruits. J. Agric. Food Chem. 50: 7449–7454.)

➤ Health benefits from consumption of whole plant foods extend beyond lowering the risk of developing cancers, CVD, cataracts, age-related macular degeneration, central neurodegenerative diseases, and diabetes. The synergistic effects of over 5000 phytochemicals have been suggested. The current hypothesis is that many unknown phytochemicals in plant foods increase the potency of the known phytonutrients health effects for reducing disease. Research names *Phenolic* compounds found in whole plant foods responsible for potent antioxidant and anticancer effects. The known effects are observed in whole plant food nutrition, but when the same compounds are isolated, the potency effect is remarkably reduced. (Chu YF, Sun J, Wu X, Liu RH. Antioxidant and antiproliferative activities of common vegetables. J Agric Food Chem. 2002 Nov 6;50(23):6910-6;

- Sun J, Chu YF, Wu X, Liu RH. Antioxidant and antiproliferative activities of common fruits. J Agric Food Chem. 2002 Dec 4;50(25):7449-54; Sun J, Liu RH. Apple phytochemical extracts inhibit proliferation of estrogen-dependent and estrogen-independent human breast cancer cells through cell cycle modulation. J Agric Food Chem. 2008 Dec 24;56(24):11661-7.)
- Research on rats exposed to a carcinogen (Aflatoxin) consumed 20% of their calories from milk protein grew tumors, while rats eating only 5% milk protein did not grow tumors. (See: Madhavan TV, Gopalan C. The effect of dietary protein on carcinogenesis of aflatoxin. Arch Pathol. 1968 Feb;85(2):133-7.)
- Research in humans consuming 20% animal milk protein (casein) exposed to the same as #9 above carcinogen (Aflatoxin) also increased pre-cancer Foci cell growth rate, while those who consumed only 5% of this milk protein with the same carcinogen exposure did not increase pre-cancer foci cell growth. (See: Youngman LD, Campbell TC. Inhibition of aflatoxin B1-induced gamma-glutamyltranspeptidase positive (GGT+) hepatic preneoplastic foci and tumors by low protein diets: evidence that altered GGT+ foci indicate neoplastic potential. Carcinogenesis. 1992 Sep;13(9):1607-13.)

➢ Researchers identified a protein fed to rats that increase in precursor foci-cancer cells. As carcinogen-exposure was kept constant in rats fed different types of proteins such as casein milk protein or plant proteins from wheat or soy. Only the carcinogen-exposed animals that consumed 20% animal-source milk protein increased precursor cancer cell production. Rats that consumed 20% protein from plant food sources did not increase cancer cell production. (See: Schulsinger DA, Root MM, Campbell TC. Effect of dietary protein quality on development of aflatoxin B1-induced hepatic preneoplastic lesions. J Natl Cancer Inst. 1989 Aug 16;81(16):1241-5.)

➢ Research shows consuming less than 10% protein calories results in less cancers in both transgenic and carcinogen-exposed animals. When animal source milk protein calorie consumption goes above 10%, the rate of cancer increases proportionately. (See: Horio F, Youngman LD, Bell RC, Campbell TC. Thermogenesis, low-protein diets, and decreased development of AFB1-induced preneoplastic foci in rat liver. Nutr Cancer. 1991;16(1):31-41.)

➢ Harmful effects can result from eating less than 1-ounce of animal-source meats such as beef, poultry, or fish known to contain saturated fat and cholesterol absent from most plant foods. The high renal acid load resulting from meat consumption is the mechanism associated with mineral imbalances in several diseases. An increased rate of calcium loss occurs with meat consumption. Robertson reports that eating 20-grams meat increases the risk of kidney stone formation. (See: Robertson WG, Peacock M, and Hodgkinson A. "Dietary changes and in the incidence of urinary calculi in the UK between 1958 and 1976." Chron. Dis. 32 (1979): 469-476.)

➢ Animal food's protein and saturated fat content raises the risk of Type I diabetes, Lupus, rheumatoid arthritis, and MS. (Lecture TCC502, Dr. T. Colin Campbell, eCornell Plant Food Certificate Course)

➢ Researchers stated that a 5% increase in energy adjusted fat intake from meat was associated with a 21% increase in the likelihood of having one additional CVD risk factor.
(Polychronopoulos E, et al., Dietary meat fats and burden of cardiovascular disease risk factors, in the elderly: a report from the MEDIS study. Lipids Health Dis. 2010 Mar 18;9:30.)

> Scientists named a dietary link between the hormone, Insulin-like Growth Factor-1 and an increased risk of prostate cancer. Previous studies showed that levels of this hormone are higher in men who eat a lot of meat, cheese, milk and butter, while strict vegetarians have low levels. (See: Roddam AW, et al., Insulin-like growth factors, their binding proteins, and prostate cancer risk: analysis of individual patient data from 12 prospective studies. Ann Intern Med. 2008 Oct 7;149(7):461-71, W83-8.)

> Scientists concluded that as vegetable to animal protein ratio increases, the risk of osteoporosis dramatically decreases. (See: Frassetto LA, Todd KM, Morris C, Jr., et al. "World incidence of hip fracture in elderly women relation to consumption of animal and vegetable foods." J. Gerentology 55 (2000): M585-M592.

> As animal source dairy milk consumption increases so do the rates of Multiple Sclerosis and Diabetes increase. (See: Dahl-Jorgensen K, Joner G, and Hanssen KF. "Relationship between cow's milk consumption and incidence of IDDM in childhood." Diabetes Care 14 (1991): 1081-1085; Malosse D, Perron H, Sasco A, et al. "Correlation between milk and dairy product consumption and multiple sclerosis prevalence: a worldwide study." Neuroepidemiology 11 (1992): 304-312.)

➢ A proposal for food-focused research might build the knowledge base for etiologic discovery and appropriate dietary advice. The diet-heart disease dilemma is put forward as an example of where a nutrient-based approach has limitations, and a summary of studies targeting food composition strengthens the case for a food-based approach. (Jacobs DR, Gallaher DD. Whole grain intake and cardiovascular disease: a review. Curr Atheroscler Rep 2004;6:415–23.)

➢ One review argues for shifting the focus towards food in order to better understand the nutrition-health interface. It begins by introducing the concept of food synergy (a perspective that more information can be obtained by looking at foods than at single food components) to denote the action of the food matrix (the composite of naturally occurring food components) on human biological systems. There are many examples confirming food synergy. More examples involved plant foods such as whole grain, apples, tomatoes, pomegranates, and broccoli. (Jacobs DR, Tapsell LC. Food, not nutrients, is the fundamental unit in nutrition. Nutr Rev 2007;65:439–50.)

> Epidemiological and prospective studies indicate that comprehensive lifestyle changes may modify the gene expression-progression of prostate cancer. Ornish and colleagues examined what would happen to gene expression in 30 men with low-risk prostate cancer by their eating a plant food diet and exercising. In 90-days, this group recorded 48 genes turned on and 452 genes turned off. This was concluded that nutrition and lifestyle change may modulate gene expression in the prostate for effective prevention and treatment. (Ornish D, Magbanua MJ, Weidner G, Weinberg V, Kemp C, Green C, Mattie MD, Marlin R, Simko J, Shinohara K, Haqq CM, Carroll PR. Changes in prostate gene expression in men undergoing an intensive nutrition and lifestyle intervention. Proc Natl Acad Sci U S A. 2008 Jun 17;105(24):8369-74. Epub 2008 Jun 16.)

Conclusion

These 21 summary statements argue that a combination of nutrients found in whole plant foods contribute to health while eating animal foods is associated with compromised health. The synergy-good effect from whole plant foods far exceeds the effects observed when a single nutrient is supplemented.[103] Nevertheless, when a deficient nutrient is replaced, compromised health may be completely restored. One Scientist stated, "900 phytonutrients have been identified as components of food." [104] Future estimates predict discovery of as many as 40,000 phytochemicals from whole plant foods [105].

---

[103] The "Synergy Effect from this large number of nutrients in whole plant foods may be the mechanism to resolve disease and spurn vigorous health.

[104] Disease-Fighting Phytonutrients, Linda Antinoro, R.D., L.D.N., J.D., C.D.E., Brigham and Women's Hospital, Previously published on Intelihealth.com, May 23, 2003. See:

Chapter VIII FOODS FOR ENERGY

Most of us always want more energy. Look at all the caffeinated drinks and energy bars on supermarket shelves. Is it possible that a dietary protocol would generate a performance-enhancing effect? Professional and Olympic athletes are tested regularly to determine if they have been using prohibited performance-enhancing substances that will generate more *energy from three pathways*:

1. **Optimal lean muscle mass anabolic growth**
2. **Enhanced oxygen transfer**
3. **Modulated metabolic hormone effects**

Cornell University Nutrition Scientist, Professor T. Colin Campbell, best-selling author, proposes that a whole plant food (vegan diet) will significantly improve each of these metabolic pathways for increasing energy performance. [106] [107]

1. **– Plant Food Diet improves lean muscle mass to fat mass ratio (BMI) and increases metabolism (BMR).**[108] Campbell compared the average calorie intake of 2640 k/cal in China (from plant-foods) associated with their lean body mass index, 21.0.

---

http://www.brighamandwomens.org/healtheweightforwomen/special_topics/phytonutrients.pdf

[105] Doug DiPasquale, Author, Holistic Nutritionist, "Phytonutrients: What Exactly Are They?" @
http://www.thatsfit.ca/2009/04/08/phytonutrients-what-exactly-are-they/

[106] Campbell TC. Campbell TM. *The China Study*. Benbella Books. Dallas, Texas.

[107] Intervention application time is 40-180 days for effect.

[108] BMI stands for Body Mass Index and BMR for Basal Metabolic Rate.

2. Campbell compared American's calorie intake of 1980 k/cal per day with their obese body mass index, 27.0. Vegan-source calories appear to generate a higher basal metabolic rate (BMR) than animal-source calories. Researchers found that rats fed vegetarian-only calories (or a diet of 95% Vegan + 5% animal-protein) exercised 200% more revolutions counted on training wheels as compared to rats eating a high protein non-vegan diet.[109] Poehlman (1988) reported that humans (vegetarians) have higher metabolic rates compared to those whose diets consist of animal-source calories.[110] Evidence of this higher basal metabolic rate (BMR) is observed in weight loss recorded in subjects shortly after they changed from animal-source calories to a whole plant food menu (below). [111] Vegetarians metabolize calories at a higher basal metabolic rate than those eating animal-based foods, resulting in weight loss and lower Body Mass Index (BMI):

WHOLE PLANT FOOD EFFECT ON BMI & WEIGHT LOSS

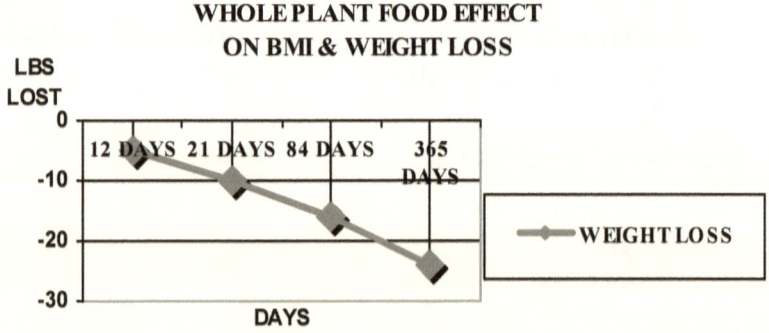

[109] Kreiger E., Youngman LD., Campbell TC., "The modulation of Aflatoxin (AFB1) – induced preneoplastic lesions by dietary protein and voluntary exercise in fischer rates. FASEB J. 2 (1988): 3304 abs.
[110] Poehlman ET., Arciero PJ., Melby CL. et al. "Resting metabolic rate and postprandial thermogensis in vegetarians and nonvegetrarians." Am J. Clin. Nutr. 48 (1988): 209-213.
[111] Campbell TC. Campbell TM. *The China Study*. Benbella Books. Dallas, Texas. pp 139.

Weight loss occurs in subjects eating 30% more calories from plant foods while those consuming less animal-source calories typically experience weight gain issues. We are what we eat and to a large extent: food choice-calories contribute to either positive or negative effect on body mass. Lean Body Mass Index is associated with whole plant foods effect on increasing basal metabolism rate.

Campbell discovered that a whole plant food menu (China) effectively reduces total body mass index (BMI) comparing Chinese dietary habits to the typical American animal foods.[112] The Chinese, who average a BMI of 21.0, eat mostly whole plant foods and eat 1/3rd more calories than Americans whose average BMI is an obese 27.0. That one may eat more calories yet have a lower BMI may mean metabolism is effected by the type of foods consumed. [113] For the moment consider the body-mass performance advantage for a cyclist climbing up a hill with a lean 21.0 BMI against an obese rider whose BMI is 27.0.

The graphic illustration on the next page shows how what we eat affects both BMI and metabolism:

---

[112] Campbell TC. Campbell TM. *The China Study.* Benbella Books. Dallas, Texas. pp 74.
[113] Ibid. Taken from a survey of 2400 counties of 880 million citizens of China.

CHINA LOW BMI FROM PLANT FOODS COMPARED TO USA HIGH BMI FROM ANIMAL FOODS

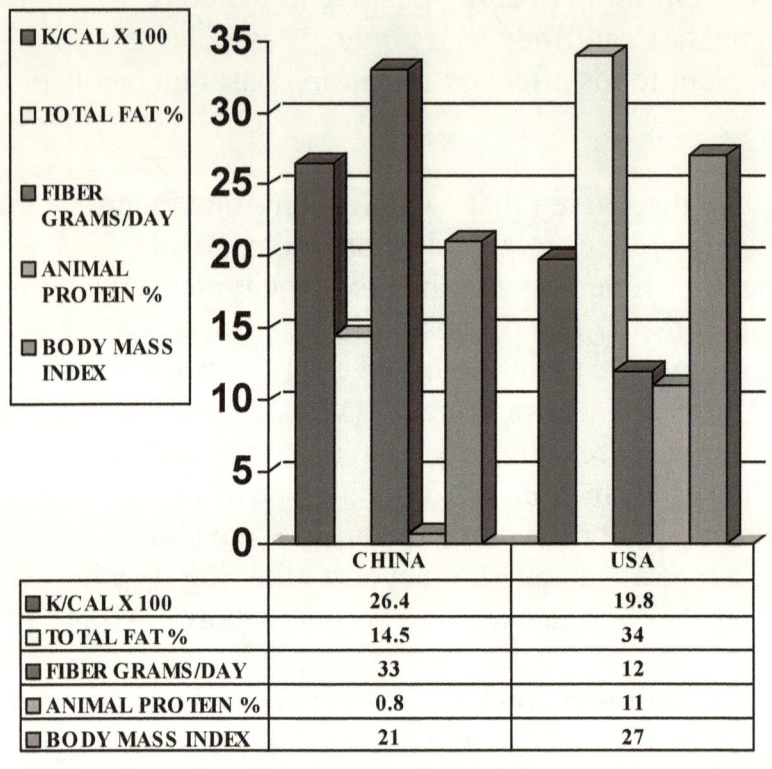

	CHINA	USA
■ K/CAL X 100	26.4	19.8
□ TOTAL FAT %	14.5	34
■ FIBER GRAMS/DAY	33	12
▨ ANIMAL PROTEIN %	0.8	11
▨ BODY MASS INDEX	21	27

2. The whole plant food diet improves blood oxygen transfer rate, prevents, and reverses heart disease.

Cardiovascular blood flow dynamics are of interest to athletes and cardio-pathological patients. Blood flow and oxygen carrying capacity can be hindered by coronary artery disease progression. The athlete's exercise proficiency is not immune from the harmful effect of poor dietary choices associated with coronary artery disease. The progression of coronary artery disease inhibits both blood flow rate and energy performance. Esselstyn reported that a whole plant food diet (appropriately applied 32-60 months) reversed progressive coronary artery disease in human subjects: [114] [115]

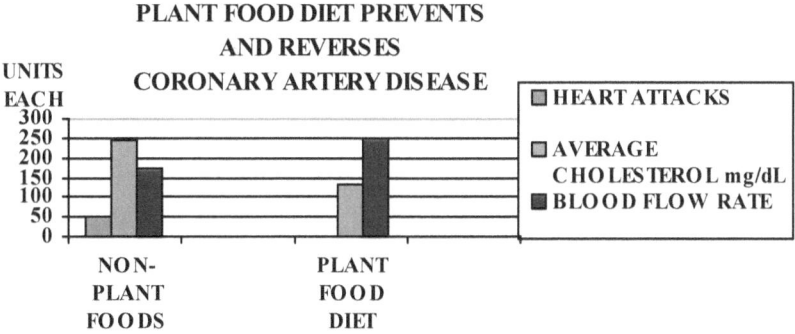

When a plant food diet is strictly adhered to, coronary artery disease is reversed. Esselstyn demonstrated this with these remarkable angiograms one, <u>before</u> "A" and one <u>after</u> "B" from a subject after 32-months strict compliance to a plant-food diet: [116]

---

[114] "A" picture is 90% blocked, after 32-months on the vegan diet, picture "B" is 100% has no blockage.

[115] Esselstyn CB. Ellis SB. Medendorps SV. et al. "A strategy to arrest and reverse coronary artery disease: a 5-year longitudinal study of a single physician's practice." J Family Practice 41 (1995): 560-568.

[116] Ibid.

Picture #1 - Coronary angiograms of the distal left anterior descending artery before (A) and after (B) 32-months of a plant-based diet without cholesterol-lowering medication prove profound improvement:

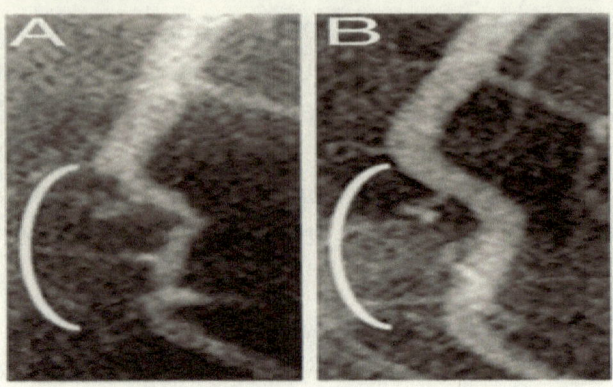

Therefore the whole plant food diet is associated with an anti-atherosclerosis effect. Atherosclerosis is associated with a reduced blood flow oxygen carrying capacity whose end result is death. Atherosclerosis is prevented by a plant food diet. Where a plant food menu is consumed, the death rate decreases and survivor rates increase. Where a whole plant food diet is not consumed, the death rate increase and survivors decrease. Morrison confirmed these dietary associations by comparing the death rates associated with how much plant food was consumed over an 8-year period. He showed that survival rate was remarkably higher in those consuming a plant food diet compared to those who did not: [117]

---

[117] Morrison LM. "Diet in atherosclerosis." JAMA (1960): 884-888.

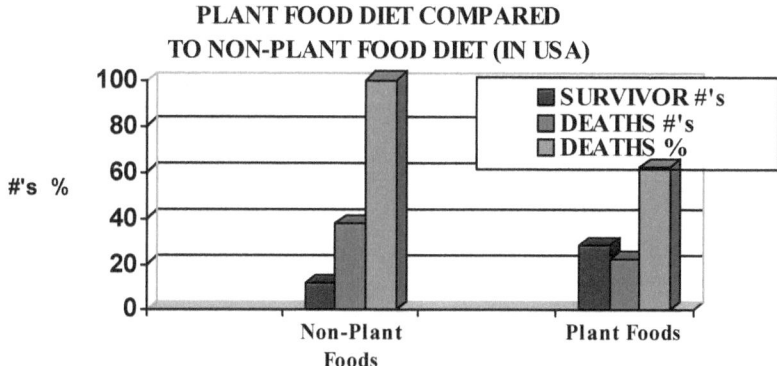

PLANT FOOD DIET COMPARED
TO NON-PLANT FOOD DIET (IN USA)

3. A plant food diet improves blood glucose efficiency, prevents, or reverses diabetes. Hinsworth reported (1935) that in countries where plant-foods are consumed most (Japan), death from diabetes occurs less as compared to other countries (USA) where animal-foods are consumed most: [118]

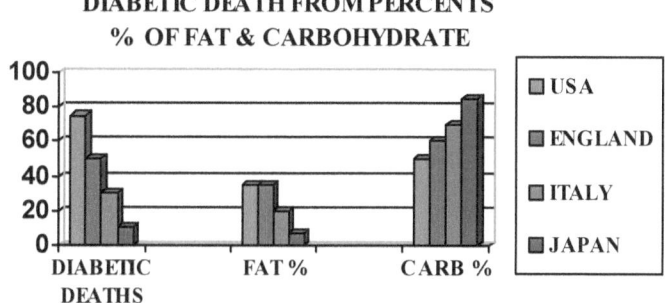

DIABETIC DEATH FROM PERCENTS
% OF FAT & CARBOHYDRATE

---

[118] Hinsworth HP. "Diet and the incidence of Diabetes Mellitus. Clin Sci 2 (1935): 117-148."

CONCLUSION

There is no question regarding the academic importance of plant foods and their potential effect on human health. When a plant food diet is added to a regular exercise training schedule, an increase in lean muscle mass to fat mass ratio, an increase in cardiovascular blood oxygen flow, an increase in basal metabolic rate BMR, a hormone-modulated improved blood glucose efficiency, and a significant decrease in total fat mass are considered performance-enhancing effects realized from increased energy.

WHOLE PLANT FOODS FOR INCREASED ENERGY What do I do?

Strict adherence to a plant food diet emphasizes avoiding animal source calories. Lack of compliance from consuming animal source foods inhibits attaining these benefits.

➢ Animal food calories ⬇ depress metabolism and stimulate weight gain +30% ⬆.

➢ Plant food calories metabolize 30% ⬆ higher than animal source calories resulting in an increase in metabolism and a need to consume more calories.

➢ Consume a minimum of 1400 calories daily from a variety of plant foods to insure adequate but not excess protein. Consuming more calories from plant foods insures adequate energy levels.

➢ Weight loss ⬇ and blood sugar balance ⇄ occurs as early as 21-days consuming a plant food diet.

➢ Total reduction ⬇ of cardiovascular accumulated plaque-buildup is attained in 30-60 months.

➢ Energy gain ⬆ creates a dynamic need to spend energy through some form of activity or exercise.

- A number of well-known athletes consume a whole plant food diet and have attained world-class performances: Sean Yates, Professional cyclist (Tour de France stage winner), Brendan Brazier, Professional Ironman triathlete, Dave Scott, Six-time winner of the Ironman triathlon, Ruth Heidrich, Six-time Ironwoman, USA track and field Master's champion, Cheryl Marek & Estelle Gray. World record holders, cross-country tandem cycling, Sixto Linares, World record holder, 24-hour triathlon, Scott Jurek, Ultramarathoner, Course Record Holder at Badwater and Western States, Debbie Lawrence, World record holder, women's 5K racewalk, Ben Matthews, U.S. Master's marathon champion, Bill Pickering, World record-holding swimmer, Jane Wetzel, U.S. National marathon champion, Robert Sweetgall, World Champion ultradistance walker, Liisa Veijalainen, World Champion orienteerer, Paavo Nurmi, considered the greatest track and field athlete of all time, long-distance runner, competed in the 1920, 1924, 1928 Olympics, winning 12 Olympic medals.
- Chris Campbell, wrestler, at age 37, won a bronze medal at the 1992 Olympics, becoming the oldest American to medal in Olympic wrestling, Carl Lewis, won 10 Olympic medals, including 9 golds, in a career that spanned from 1979 to 1996, competing for the USA, Debbie Lawrence, racewalker & three-time Olympian (1992, 1996, and 2000) is the world record holder for the women's 5K racewalk event.

➢ The plant food lifestyle is recommended for a minimum of 90-days to attain the positive benefits of increased energy, enhanced vascular blood flow volume, circulating blood sugars balance, with significant loss of body fat weight.

CHAPTER IX DIETARY SUPPLEMENTS

Supplement nutrient deficiency justifies dose. What nutrients should be supplemented with the whole plant food lifestyle? Because eating a variety of whole plant foods supplies as few as 900 phytonutrient substances (known) [119] to as many as 40,000 phytonutrients (upper estimate, yet to be discovered), [120] very little supplementation to replace deficiencies is needed. Several colleagues, Alternative Medicine Physicians, Nutritionists, and Naturopaths report more of patients' health issues are caused by supplement overdose than from deficiency. People have a mindset that, "If some supplements are good, then more is better." Supplement overdose results in unexplained health issues often resolved by taking patient off supplements completely.

Nevertheless, a plant food menu may be low in iron, zinc, vitamin B12, omega-3 fatty acids, vitamin D, calcium, and iodine. [121] Supplement dosage is justified by diagnostic tests. Taking supplemental Vitamin D 2000-5000 iu per day when sunlight exposure is limited, omega-3 from ground flax seed (1 tablespoon/day), and sublingual Vitamin B12 (100-200 micrograms/day) are supplements to consider adding to a diet of whole plant foods. Typically, adding these nutrients at these doses will not cause an overdose reaction.

---

[119] Disease-Fighting Phytonutrients, Linda Antinoro, R.D., L.D.N., J.D., C.D.E., Brigham and Women's Hospital, Previously published on Intelihealth.com, May 23, 2003. See: http://www.brighamandwomens.org/healtheweightforwomen/special_topics/phytonutr ients.pdf

[120] Doug DiPasquale, Author, Holistic Nutritionist, "Phytonutrients: What Exactly Are They?" @ http://www.thatsfit.ca/2009/04/08/phytonutrients-what-exactly-are-they/

[121] Key TJ, Appleby PN, Rosell MS: "Health effects of vegetarian and vegan diets" (abstract). Proceedings of the Nutrition Society, 2006, 65:35-41.

The required RDA Nutrient dose question may be stated, "Nutrient deficiency justifies dose." What required nutrient dose prevents deficiency? From the years 1995-2010, I computer-analyzed (via the

First Data Bank Nutritionist Pro IV dietary analysis software) the actual weighed food-intake of 70 subjects. Each food item was weighed prior to being consumed. From these diets, I was not able to detect a single one that provided the "Required Daily Allowance (RDA)" for all vitamins and/or all minerals we are told we need daily. From the diets analyzed, I chose 10 men and 10 women that contained the most foods consumed each day. Of those 20 subjects no one list foods consumed provided 100% of the RDA vitamin-minerals required. This paper was subsequently peer-reviewed and published in the Journal of the International Society of Sports Nutrition. [122]

If food intake fails to provide the required nutrients, is it possible that some health issues may be attributed to prolonged nutrient deficiencies? Of the 10 men's and 10 women's diets analyzed, RDA-deficiency ranged from 3-14 nutrients under the "required" 10 vitamins or 7 minerals. Since the subject's food intake did not supply the RDA-requirement for all nutrients, why were they so healthy? This begs two questions:
1. Is the RDA-nutrient requirement an accurate tool to justify supplement dose?
2. Why were no health issues associated with a nutrient deficiency in the subjects measured in this study?

---

[122] Misner B. Food alone may not provide sufficient micronutrients for preventing deficiency. J Int Soc Sports Nutr. 2006 Jun 5;3:51-5. PubMed PMID: 18500963; PubMed Central PMCID: PMC2129155. @
http://www.ncbi.nlm.nih.gov/pmc/articles/PMC2129155/?tool=pubmed

MICRONUTRIENT	MEN % Reference Daily Intake (RDI)					WOMEN % Reference Daily Intake (RDI)				
MALE (M) WOMEN (W) ACTIVE (A) SEDENTARY (S)	M1 (A)	M2 (A)	M3 (S)	M4 (A)	M5 (A)	W1 (A)	W2 (A)	W3 (A)	W4 (A)	W5 (A)
TOTAL CALORIES INTAKE REPORTED	55%	59%	53%	161%	112%	64%	77%	138%	104%	103%
VITAMIN A	71%	116%	69%	445%	49%	241%	1617%	203%	95%	807%
VITAMIN D	19%	59%	63%	30%	32%	10%	38%	1%	70%	8%
VITAMIN E	43%	135%	18%	76%	66%	146%	95%	154%	64%	206%
VITAMIN K	19%	311%	11%	122%	61%	18%	511%	44%	78%	155%
VITAMIN B-1	71%	103%	140%	290%	183%	64%	168%	334%	389%	264%
VITAMIN B-2	69%	95%	67%	209%	342%	77%	146%	183%	382%	183%
VITAMIN B-3	155%	87%	64%	294%	123%	117%	267%	256%	270%	214%
VITAMIN B-6	90%	144%	55%	137%	77%	81%	231%	143%	180%	213%
VITAMIN B-12	99%	156%	123%	193%	357%	119%	140%	78%	99%	328%
FOLATE	55%	235%	76%	255%	233%	73%	130%	249%	174%	311%
IODINE	0%	58%	0%	0%	36%	0%	25%	31%	0%	58%
POTASSIUM	124%	212%	67%	253%	144%	94%	206%	217%	201%	238%
CALCIUM	53%	90%	77%	179%	111%	65%	84%	118%	182%	99%
MAGNESIUM	51%	124%	44%	175%	73%	82%	140%	207%	119%	156%
PHOSPHORUS	105%	169%	138%	175%	248%	89%	113%	411%	218%	249%
ZINC	35%	55%	48%	124%	97%	35%	78%	144%	67%	164%
SELENIUM	30%	44%	24%	159%	97%	3%	120%	256%	117%	174%
INDIVIDUAL MICRONUTRIENT DEFICIENCIES	14	7	15	3	9	13	5	4	7	3

TABLE 2.
Group I (5 Men, 5 Women)

TABLE 3.
Group II (5 MEN, 5 WOMEN)

MICRONUTRIENT	MEN % Reference Daily Intake (RDI)					WOMEN % Reference Daily Intake (RDI)				
MALE (M) WOMEN (W)	M6 (S)	M7 (A)	M8 (A)	M9 (A)	M10 (A)	W6 (A)	W7 (S)	W8 (S)	W9 (S)	W10 (S)
TOTAL CALORIES INTAKE REPORTED	42%	161%	56%	93%	134%	125%	118%	76%	104%	64%
VITAMIN A	248%	445%	105%	129%	117%	533%	318%	326%	216%	130%
VITAMIN D	75%	30%	66%	13%	125%	86%	43%	60%	6%	16%
VITAMIN E	1%	76%	0.2%	123%	93%	19%	195%	9%	173%	39%
VITAMIN K	205%	122%	104%	95%	73%	341%	110%	197%	189%	28%
VITAMIN B-1	101%	290%	95%	137%	187%	255%	206%	98%	176%	155%
VITAMIN B-2	100%	209%	106%	167%	189%	219%	191%	113%	143%	84%
VITAMIN B-3	119%	294%	126%	130%	198%	204%	207%	163%	186%	167%
VITAMIN B-6	97%	137%	73%	117%	167%	168%	141%	125%	133%	128%
VITAMIN B-12	146%	193%	179%	216%	224%	111%	191%	182%	161%	98%
FOLATE	151%	255%	137%	190%	260%	327%	156%	131%	209%	171%
IODINE	0%	0%	18%	0%	0%	0%	0%	0%	0%	0%
POTASSIUM	136%	253%	99%	137%	260%	206%	135%	171%	122%	73%
CALCIUM	59%	179%	77%	127%	193%	178%	95%	103%	114%	69%
MAGNESIUM	75%	175%	72%	92%	146%	167%	125%	110%	130%	77%
PHOSPHORUS	119%	321%	135%	193%	254%	213%	148%	149%	144%	65%
ZINC	41%	124%	71%	68%	96%	98%	98%	67%	63%	56%
SELENIUM	55%	159%	47%	74%	122%	125%	85%	173%	146%	115%
INDIVIDUAL MICRONUTRIENT DEFICIENCIES	8	3	10	6	4	4	5	5	3	11

TABLE 4. MICRONUTRIENT DEFICITS			
MICRONUTRIENT	MICRONUTRIENT RDA Deficiency %	MEN NUMBER DEFICIT	WOMEN NUMBER DEFICIT
IODINE[123]	100%	10	10
VITAMIN D	95%	9	10
ZINC	80%	8	8
VITAMIN E	65%	8	5
CALORIES	50%	6	4
CALCIUM	50%	5	5
SELENIUM	45%	7	2
VITAMIN K	45%	5	4
MAGNESIUM	40%	6	2
VITAMIN B-6	30%	5	1
VITAMIN B-2	25%	3	2
VITAMIN A	25%	3	2
VITAMIN B-1	20%	2	2
VITAMIN B-12	20%	1	3
POTASSIUM	20%	2	2
FOLATE	15%	2	1
VITAMIN B-3	10%	2	0
PHOSPHORUS	10%	0	2

---

[123] Iodine is present in sea vegetation, but not in most foods unless iodized salt is added. An iodine intake of less than 20 micrograms (ug) per day is considered severe deficiency; 20-50 micrograms (ug) per day is considered moderate deficiency and 50-100 micrograms (ug) per day are considered mild deficiency. Iodized salt is widely used and some other foods are fortified with iodine. Two grams of iodized salt supplies 150 micrograms (0.15 mg). None of the dietary analysis included NaCl added by the consumer to food. This may an inaccurate estimate of the iodine deficiency rate.

Dr. Matt Lederman, a board-certified internist who specializes in nutrition and lifestyle medicine, asked this important question:

"The RDA of vitamins and minerals is based on population studies and how much people require of a particular nutrient to keep the population from exhibiting deficiency symptoms. You may not be the typical American they used in determining the RDA. You may be following a healthy, low-fat, plant-based diet, and with such an optimized diet and lifestyle, your body may thrive on less. In fact, when your vitamin D level is optimized, you can absorb twice as much calcium from a particular meal as someone with insufficient vitamin D levels. At that point, excess calcium supplementation actually impairs vitamin D conversion and causes more trouble than good. So someone with a normal vitamin D level requires much less calcium than someone with an insufficient or deficient vitamin D level. There are many examples like this, where one vitamin or mineral affects the absorption of other vitamins and minerals." [124]

Dr. Lederman's point is that each person has a specific nutrient need, which is precisely controlled by internal mechanisms. This may mean that science should review the accuracy of the current DRI/RDA-nutrient dose.

---

[124] TCC503 from Dr. Matt Lederman's Lecture, by permission, courtesy of eCornell Plant Food Certificate Course @: http://www.tcolincampbell.org/courses-resources/

Nutrient Deficiency Deserves Dose (replacement)

If a health issue is associated with deficiency of calcium, iodine, iron, or zinc, diagnostic testing should be ordered to determine deficiency for replenishing deficiency and restoring health.

Nutrient Deficiency Deserves Dose (replacement)		
Nutrient	RDA Daily Dose	Deficiency Test
Iodine	US Institute of Medicine (IOM) recommended dietary allowance (RDA) is 150 mcg/d of iodine for adults and adolescents. Iodine Deficiency Disorder (IDD) in a population is a median 24-hour urine iodine collection. If a 24-hour urine collection is not practical, a random urine iodine-to-creatinine ratio can be used instead. In this case, a median of 50-100 mcg of iodine per liter is consistent with mild iodine deficiency, 20-49 mcg of iodine per liter is consistent with moderate deficiency, and less than 20 mcg of iodine per liter is consistent with severe deficiency.	Physician-ordered Iodine/Iodide loading test is based on the concept that the normally functioning human body has a mechanism to retain ingested iodine until whole body sufficiency for iodine is determined by a negative feedback mechanism triggered to adjust excretion of iodine to balance the intake. As iodine content increases, the iodine load percent % retained decreases with an increase in amount of iodide excreted in the 24-hour urine collection.
Calcium	1000-1300 milligrams/day* *Best consumed from whole plant food sources [avoid supplemental Calcium].	Physician-ordered CBC, urinalysis, chemistry panel, 24-hr urine calcium, PTH assay, serum protein electrophoresis, serum 25-OH vitamin D3 , skeletal survey, bone scan, d -xylose absorption test, serum 1,25-(OH) 2 vitamin D, and an endocrinology consult should be considered in the workup.
Zinc	8-14 milligrams per day	The optimal range of plasma zinc is 13.8-22.9µmol/L (90-150µg/dl). Clinical signs of zinc deficiency may occur when plasma zinc concentrations drop below 9.9µmol/L (65 µg/dl). Values less than 5µmol/L (33 µg/dl) are particularly associated with loss of the senses of taste and smell, abdominal pain, diarrhea, skin rash, and loss of appetite. A 10-second test that uses a dilute solution of zinc sulphate heptahydrate to determine the extent of zinc deficiency based on an individual's taste sensations.
Iron (Precaution: Do not take iron supplements without Physician monitored treatment.)	Males 14-18 years old - 15 milligrams per day Females 14-18 years old - 18 milligrams per day Males 19-50 years old - 8 milligrams per day	Physician-monitored tests are ordered to measure iron levels. These tests can show how much iron has been used from body's stored iron. Three tests include: (1) Serum iron. This test measures the amount of iron in blood. The level of iron in blood may be normal even if the total amount of iron in the body is low. For this reason, other iron tests also are ordered:

	Females 19-50 years old - 18 milligrams per day Males and females 51 years and older, 8 milligrams per day Pregnant females all ages, 27 milligrams per day Lactating females age 14-18, 10 milligrams per day Lactating females over age 19, 9 milligrams per day Precaution: Do not take iron supplements without Physician monitored prescription assistance.	(2) Serum ferritin. Ferritin is a protein that helps store iron in the body. A measure of this protein helps the doctor find out how much of the body's stored iron is depleted. (3) Transferrin level or total iron-binding capacity. Transferrin is a protein that carries iron in the blood. Total iron-binding capacity measures how much of the transferrin in blood isn't carrying iron. If iron-deficiency anemia presents, a high level of transferrin that has no iron results.
Vitamin B12	The Dietary Reference Intake for an adult ranges from 2-3 micrograms μg per day. Vitamin B12 supplements are safe when used orally in amounts that do not exceed the recommended dietary allowance (RDA). The Physicians Committee for Responsible Medicine recommends that vegans either consistently eat foods fortified with B12 or take a daily or weekly B12 supplement. Adults age 51 and older are recommended to consume B12 fortified food or supplements to meet the RDA, because they are at an increased risk for deficiency. [125]	Laboratory tests are physician-ordered to diagnose and monitor B12 and Folate deficiency: B12. If low, a deficiency is indicated, but it does not identify the cause. If normal, a Folate deficiency may be present. May be ordered to monitor the effectiveness of treatment. (2) CBC (Complete Blood Count). A group of tests ordered routinely to screen for blood cell abnormalities. It measures cell types, quantities, and characteristics. With both B12 and Folate deficiency anemia, the amount of hemoglobin may be low and the red blood cells (RBCs) are abnormally large (macrocytic or megaloblastic). White blood cells and platelets also may be decreased. (3) Folate. Either serum or RBC folate may be tested. Some believe that the RBC-Folate is more clinically relevant. If either is low, a deficiency is indicated. If normal, a B12 deficiency may still be present and may be ordered to monitor the effectiveness of treatment.
Vitamin D	Birth-18 years 5 mcg 19-50 years 5 mcg 51-70 years 10 mcg 71+ years 15 mcg (200 IU = 5 mcg) (400 IU = 10 mcg) (600 IU = 15 mcg)	Physician monitored 1-2-3 tests for Vitamin D are as follows: (1) 25-hydroxyvitamin D. If calcium is low or the patient has symptoms of vitamin D deficiency, such as bone malformation in children (rickets) and bone weakness, softness, or fracture in adults (osteomalacia), 25-hydroxyvitamin D usually is ordered to identify a possible deficiency in vitamin D. Vitamin D deficiency is thought to be much more common than previously

---

[125] "Don't Vegetarians Have Trouble Getting Enough Vitamin B12?". Physicians Committee for Responsible Medicine. http://www.pcrm.org/health/veginfo/b12.html

		believed. Some studies have shown as many as 50% of the elderly and women being treated for osteoporosis are Vitamin D deficient. 25-hydroxyvitamin D is often ordered before an individual begins drug therapy for osteoporosis. Some osteoporosis medications now include the recommended Vitamin D dose. (2) 1,25-dihydroxyvitamin D. If calcium is high or the patient has a disease that may produce excess amounts of vitamin D, such as sarcoidosis or some forms of lymphoma, 1,25-dihydroxyvitamin D test usually is ordered. Rarely, this testing is indicated when abnormalities of 1-alphahydroxylase are suspect. (3) Vitamin D levels also may be used to help diagnose or monitor problems with parathyroid gland functioning since PTH is essential for vitamin D activation. When vitamin D, calcium, phosphorus, or magnesium supplementation is necessary, vitamin D levels are sometimes measured to monitor treatment effectiveness.
Omega-3	Males 1.6 g/day Females 1.1 g/day *Best source is whole plant foods walnuts, flaxseeds. [Avoid supplemental sources.]	No standardized test is identified for Omega-3.

To attain optimal health and avoid the potential risk of nutrient deficiency, eat a variety of colored whole plant foods [next page].

.

Colored Plant Foods – More Colors = Better Health

Eating a variety of Green, Red, Orange, Blue, Purple, and White whole plant foods supplies most nutrients well above the "required" (RDA/DRI) levels:

Top Foods Nutrient Profile Identified By Color		
Color	Foods	Nutrients
Red	Apples, Beets, Cherries, Cranberries, Red Grapes, Red Peppers, Pomegranates, Raspberries, Strawberries, Tomatoes, & Watermelon.	Antioxidants Anthocyanins Lycopene
Orange-Yellow	Yellow apples, Apricots, Cantaloupe, Carrots, Mangoes, Papayas, Peaches, Yellow peppers, Pumpkin, Sweet potatoes, Yellow tomatoes, & Yellow watermelon.	Antioxidants Carotenoids Vitamin A Vitamin C Folate
Green	Artichokes, Asparagus, Green beans, Broccoli, Brussels sprouts, Honeydew melon, Kale, Kiwi, Green onions, Peas, Green pepper, & Spinach	Antioxidants Indoles Lutein Folate Zeaxanthin
Blue-Purple	Blackberries, Blueberries, Figs, Plums, Prunes, Purple grapes, & Raisins.	Antioxidants Anthocyanins
Light Pale/White	Bananas, Cauliflower, Garlic, Mushrooms, Onions, Parsnips, Potatoes, Turnips	Antioxidants Allicin Potassium

Author's Note: After reviewing 70 subjects and not finding a single subject whose dietary intake provided 100% of the all the RDA/DRI daily required allowances, I question whether the nutrient requirement dosage "one-size-fits-all" medium is an accurate measure. If none are getting their daily-required nutrients, why are we not more of us suffering from deficiency diseases? I have observed persons lower total cholesterol levels, increase energy, and enjoy vigorous health simply by limiting their nutrient intake to a variety of multi-colored whole plant foods. None of these subjects attained benefits by adding dietary supplements. Limited to these observations, a diet with adequate calories from a variety of whole multi-colored plant foods provides all the nutrients and reduces the need to take a dietary supplement.

What Supplements?

1. Eat a variety of red, orange-yellow, green, blue-purple, and pale plant foods and consider the supplements listed below with your healthcare practitioner:
2. Vitamin B12 @ 200-600 micrograms/day
3. Omega-3 @ 1-2 grams from ground flax seeds/day
4. Vitamin D @ 2000-5000 iu/day (persons in Northern latitudes when sunlight exposure is limited
5. Supplement dose should be confirmed by physician-monitored diagnostic test associated with a health issue

CHAPTER X MAKING THE CHOICE
DECISIONS, DECISIONS, DECISIONS

The real merits for this dietary lifestyle described in, "Phytonutrients: Finding Fitness for Life," requires application. Whatever is decided, to do or not to do, specific consequences and rewards should be considered. The consequences associated with eating animal-derived foods are, in my opinion, a trigger mechanism responsible for several diseases associated with premature death. Consuming animal-source foods are likely to contribute to: (1) Cardiovascular plaque-clogging sequences, (2) Progression of DNA-cellular mutagenic reactions, and (3) Inflammatory reactions associated with autoimmune diseases.

The potential rewards from a whole plant food lifestyle are:
1. Reverse Cardiovascular disease
2. Reverse Cancer disease
3. Reverse Diabetes
4. Reverse Immune system diseases

However, this statement is does not suggest that dietary lifestyle by itself will reverse all forms of disease. Resolving some healthcare issues may require medical treatment in addition to dietary modifications. While the whole plant food lifestyle has been observed to reverse diseases of a large number of patients, treatment of some acute or chronic diseases may also require a Physician's allopathic intervention. After hearing all the arguments against adopting a whole plant food lifestyle, persons who apply this dietary lifestyle typically state, "I was not sure if I could do it, but now, I wished that I had done this long ago!" I have observed at or near 100% of the people who adopt eating a whole plant foods menu lose a significant amount of bodyweight (10-30 lbs) and lower their total cholesterol (50-100 points). In fact, after 90-days of eating only whole plant foods, I lost around 10 lbs bodyweight and my cholesterol decreased from 232 to 151 mg/dL. To eat only whole plant foods for 90-days is your decision. You must be absolutely persuaded in order to complete this task. This means **NO fats, NO oils, NO meats, NO milk/dairy, NO seeds/nuts for 90-days.**

You may find that after 30-days, there will be a temptation to returning to a mixed diet of part plant food with part animal foods. Any compromise permitting processed sweets or high fat foods provokes dietary habit associated with a potential health issue. This decision requires making whole plant food diet a priority for 90-days.

This decision requires removing all animal source foods from your home and is confirmed by your signature on the following pages:

AGREEMENT

After studious review of each section in *Phytonutrition: Finding Fitness For Life*, I determine the facts presented support the hypothesis that a whole plant food lifestyle prevents many diseases and restores vigorous health. I conclude this evidence supports application.

I hereby affix my signature, dated, pledging to consume a whole plant food menu for 90-days:

_____ (SIGNATURE INDICATES AGREEMENT FOR A
_____
90-DAY TRIAL)

_____

DATE SIGNED

_____

DATE 90-DAYS

Pre-test body weight: _____
Post-test body weight: _____
Pre-test body cholesterol: _____
Post-test body cholesterol: _____
Pre-test energy scale 1-10 (1 = Lowest;
10=highest):_____
Post-test energy scale 1-10 (1 = Lowest;
10=highest):_____

CHAPTER XI RECIPES
[Plant Foods That Taste Great!]

Conversion to a whole plant food menu requires time for adoption because learned tastes for fats and sugars require 30-90 days abstinence to unlearn. Once the conversion is complete, people say, "I was completely surprised how great plant foods taste!" Previously we learned that human appetite (taste) is shaped by both genetics (nature) and lifestyle (nurture). However, new taste preferences require a tincture of time for unlearning then relearning. Human taste receptors (located in the brain) are naturally attracted to calorie-dense fats, sweets, meaty (unami) flavors and textures. The denser the calorie content, the more that food is desired. Appetite, however, can be satisfied by calorie-sparse whole plant foods. Satiation requires a larger volume of plant foods to quench our natural craving for calories. Because whole plant foods are fiber–rich and calorie-sparse, the appetite is filled sooner with a bulk of fewer calories plant foods as compared to the denser calories profile found in animal source foods. Interestingly, people can eat more calories from whole plant foods than animal foods resulting in increased metabolic rate and lower body mass index. The China Study showed that the average Chinese has a slim Body Mass Index of 21, yet consumes 90% of their 2641-calories daily from whole plant foods. Conversely, the average American, who eats 1989 calories/day mostly (70%) from animal source foods, has an obese Body Mass Index of 27. (Chapter II. The China Study by T. Colin Campbell et al.)

Such results argue that we can eat more calories from plant foods to turn up metabolism and to reduce body mass index at the same time. What if we could make meals consisting of whole plant foods taste better than animal source foods?

RECIPES - Plant Foods Taste Great!
Appetites can experience sensational tastes from recipes consisting of whole plant foods. Several who have tested these recipes proclaim: "These Plant Foods Taste Great!" Each recipe is computer-analyzed (First Data Bank Nutritionist IV) to determine total fiber, total calories and the ratio of carbohydrates, protein, and fat. Some of the recipes include multiple servings with more calories than one person may eat in a single meal.

Recipe #1 Potato Bean Veggie Burgers
This recipe makes 6-8 burgers with each burger containing 7-10 grams fiber with 184-246 calories as 82% carbohydrates, 16% protein, and 2% fat. By permission, courtesy of Linda Hildebrand, Cheney, Washington.
Ingredients List: 1 can Black Beans, 1 grated carrot, ½ diced onion, 3 grated potatoes, 4 chopped scallions, 1 cup corn, 1 tsp salt, 1 tsp black pepper.
Directions: Mash beans with masher or food processor. Add remaining ingredients and shape after mixing into patties. Cook in 1 tablespoons olive oil 3 minutes on each side. Be sure to squeeze excess fluid out of grated potatoes; Substitute grated hash browns or add vegetables per taste preference.

Recipe #2 Dinosaur Kale Quinoa Wrap
This recipe contains 33 grams fiber, 1090 calories as 62% carbohydrates, 15% protein, and 23% fat.

(cont. Recipe #2 Dinosaur Kale Quinoa Wrap)…By permission, courtesy of Brendan Brazier, "THRIVE, The Vegan Nutrition Guide to Optimal Performance in Sports and Life," De Capo Press, 2008, page 241.

Ingredients List: 1 Avocado, 2 Roma Tomatoes, 1 Cucumber, 1 Carrot, 2 Strips Dulse, 1 cup soaked or cooked Quinoa, 1 leaf Dinosaur Kale, salad dressing to taste from Recipe #3.

Directions: Peel and cube avocado, slice tomatoes, slice cucumber, and grate carrot. Place along with dulse and quinoa on a leaf of kale. Drizzle salad dressing of choice (recommend recipe #3 below).

Recipe #3 Black-Eyed Pea Cayenne Salsa

This recipe contains 13 grams fiber, 361 calories as 48% carbohydrates, 16% protein, and 36% fat.

By permission, courtesy of Brendan Brazier, "THRIVE, The Vegan Nutrition Guide to Optimal Performance in Sports and Life," De Capo Press, 2008, page 265.

Ingredients List: Juice 1 lemon, 1 diced tomato, ½ diced onion, 1 cup black-eyed peas, 1 cup chopped cilantro, 1 tbsp balsalmic vinegar, 1 tbsp hemp oil, ½ tsp cayenne pepper, ½ tsp chilli flakes, ¼ tsp sea salt.

Directions: In a bowl, combine all ingredients and allow sitting for a few hours at room temperature to allow flavors to infuse. May be added to salads sandwiches or to Recipe #2 Dinosaur Kale Quinoa Wrap for flavor.

Recipe #4 Mountain Man Breakfast Cereal

This recipe makes 1-2 servings, contains 30 grams fiber, 284 calories as 71% carbohydrates, 9% protein, and 20% fat.

(cont. Recipe #4 Mountain Man Breakfast Cereal)
Ingredients List: 70 grams Quaker old fashioned rolled
oats, 16 rams organic ground flaxseeds, 20 grams psyllium
husk fiber, 1 banana, 100 grams blueberries.
Directions: Mix rolled oats, ground flaxseeds, psyllium
fiber with hot water to soften, add and stir diced banana
and blueberries. Footnote: This is a very filling cereal and
may be divided in two serving sizes.

Recipe #5 Barley Scones
This recipe makes 12 scones, contains 24 grams fiber, 637
calories as 89% carbohydrates, 8% protein, and 3% fat.
By permission, courtesy of Mike Anderson, "The RAVE
Diet & Lifestyle," www.RaveDiet.com, March 2009, page
134.
Ingredients List: 1 1/8 cup barley flour, ¼ cup water, 3
tablespoons raisins, 2 tbsp maple syrup, 1 tbsp applesauce,
2 tsp vinegar, 1 tsp baking powder, ¼ tsp baking soda.
Directions: Preheat oven to 350. Mix water, maple syrup,
applesauce and vinegar/set aside. Combine flour, baking
soda and raisins into food processor and blend. Add liquid
ingredients and process until dough forms. Transfer to flat
surface, dusted with barley flour. Flatten into a circle 6
inches in diameter and ¾ inch thick. Use knife to score
dough into 12 wedges (do not separate), and then transfer
to baking sheet. Bake for 30 minutes or until light
browned.

Recipe #6 Coffee Cake

This recipe makes 6 servings, contains 42 grams fiber, 1610 calories (268 calories per serving), 85% carbohydrate, 10% protein, and 5%.

By permission, courtesy of Mike Anderson, "The RAVE Diet & Lifestyle," www.RaveDiet.com, March 2009, page 135.

Ingredients List: 2 cups whole wheat flour, 1 cup unsweetened apple juice, ¾ cup old fashioned rolled oats, ½ cup applesauce, ½ cup maple syrup, 1 tbsp baking powder, 2 tsp cinnamon, ½ tsp ground nutmeg, ¼ tsp ginger.

Directions: Preheat oven to 350. Apply vegetable stock as an oil substitute to baking pan. In a large bowl, add flour, ½ cup oats, baking powder, cinnamon, maple syrup, nutmeg, and ginger. Remove ½ cup of mixture to a cup or small bowl, add remaining ¼ cup oats. Cut in 2 tablespoons of applesauce, set the mixture aside. Cut remaining applesauce into the flour mixture in the large bowl. Stir in the applesauce until well combined. Pour the batter into the prepared pan, Top with the reserved oat mixture. Bake about 40 minutes or until well done.

Recipe #7 The Ultimate Plant Food Meal [126]

This recipe makes 1-2 servings, contains 26 grams fiber, 454 calories (227 calories per serving), 62% carbohydrate, 23% protein, and 15 %.

Ingredients List: 89 grams black beans, 103 grams broccoli, 187 grams brussels sprouts, 118 grams diced tomatoes, 48 grams diced black olives, 88 grams spinach,

---

[126] This is my favorite, the original recipe should contain as many of the ingredients listed as raw or as individual taste tolerances allow. When consumed raw, more nutrients from food are absorbed.

(cont. Recipe #7 The Ultimate Plant Food Meal)...
54 grams green beans, 63 grams asparagus, 132 grams split pea soup with water drained, 29 grams kale leaves, 49 grams portabella mushrooms, 22 grams green onions.
Directions: Empty all ingredients into a large bowl and stir gently until mixed. Butter buds or balsamic vinegar may be added on for flavor.

Recipe #8 Black Bean and Corn
This recipe makes 3 servings, contains 76 grams fiber, 1347 calories (449 calories per serving), 75 % carbohydrate, 18% protein, and 6% fat.
By permission, courtesy of Mike Anderson, "The RAVE Diet & Lifestyle," www.RaveDiet.com, March 2009, page 143.
Ingredients List: 3 cups black beans, 2 cups corn, 2 chopped tomatoes, 1 chopped red pepper, 1 minced jalapeno pepper, 1 cup chopped green onions, ½ cup chopped onions, ½ cup chopped cilantro, 1-2 tbsp from 1 lime, 1 tbsp vegetable broth, 1 tsp minced garlic.
Directions: Combine first seven ingredients in a large bowl. Make dressing with limejuice, cilantro, garlic, pepper and vegetable broth.
Combine well. Pour over salad ingredients and toss lightly to combine. Chill several hours before serving.

Recipe #9 Italian Dressing (Salad Dressing)
This recipe makes 1 serving, contains 0.3 grams fiber, 30 calories (30 calories per serving), 85% carbohydrate, 9% protein, and 6%fat.
By permission, courtesy of Mike Anderson, "The RAVE Diet & Lifestyle," www.RaveDiet.com, March 2009, page 118.

(cont. Recipe #9 Italian Salad Dressing)… Ingredients List: Mix ¼ cup red-wine vinegar, 1 tbsp lemon juice, 1 tsp minced onion, ¼ tsp oregano, ¼ tsp basil, pinch of thyme, pinch of garlic powder.
Directions: Mix or blend thoroughly then apply to salad to suite taste.

Recipe #10 Mustard-Garlic Vinaigrette (Salad Dressing)

This recipe makes 4-cups or 8 servings (depending upon taste), contains 2 grams fiber, 157 calories (20 calories per ½ cup serving), 39% carbohydrate, 20% protein, and 41% fat.
By permission, courtesy of Mike Anderson, "The RAVE Diet & Lifestyle," www.RaveDiet.com, March 2009, page 119.
Ingredients List: Mix 2 garlic cloves, ½ cup mustard, 3 tbsp lemon juice, 3 tbsp water, 1 tsp light miso, 1 tsp low sodium Tamari soy sauce, ½ tsp maple syrup, ½ tsp curry powder.
Directions: Mix or blend thoroughly then apply to salad to suite taste.

Recipe #11 Apple Oat Muffins

This recipe makes 12 medium muffins, contains 5.25 grams fiber per muffin, 210 calories per muffin, as 86% carbohydrate, 9% protein, and 5% fat.
By permission, courtesy of Mike Anderson, "The RAVE Diet & Lifestyle," www.RaveDiet.com, March 2009, page 136.
Ingredients List: 3 cups whole wheat pastry flour, 1 apple juice concentrate12-fluid ounces, 2 finely-chopped gala or fuji apples, 1¼ cups oat bran, ½ cup raisins, 2 ½ tsp

(cont. Recipe #11 Apple Oat Muffins)…baking soda, 1 tsp ground cinnamon, ½ tsp grated/ground nutmeg.
Directions: Preheat oven to 325. In a large bowl, mix flour, oats, spices and baking soda. Add the chopped apple along with the apple juice concentrate and raisins. Stir just enough to mix. Spoon batter into muffin tins and bake for 25 minutes.

Recipe #12 Whole Wheat Pancakes
This recipe makes 24 pancakes 2"-servings, contains 1 ½ grams fiber & 23 calories per pancake serving), as 84%carbohydrate, 12 % protein, and 4% fat.
By permission, courtesy of Mike Anderson, "The RAVE Diet & Lifestyle," www.RaveDiet.com, March 2009, page 140.
Ingredients List: 1 banana, 1 ¼ cups water, 1-cup whole-wheat flour, 1 tbsp maple syrup, and 2 tsp sodium-free baking powder.
Directions: In a large bowl, mash banana, then stir in water and maple syrup. In a separate bowl, mix flour and baking powder. Add to banana mixture and stir until smooth. Pour small amounts of batter onto a preheated griddle or skillet with a small amount of oil substitutes such as any pureed fruit or apple juice. Cook until tops bubble. Flip with spatula and cook until golden brown about 1 minute. Use fresh fruit or maple syrup for serving.

Recipe #13 Aztec Salad
This recipe makes 8-cups or 4-servings, contains 15 grams fiber & 283 calories per 2-cup serving), as 75 % carbohydrate, 20% protein, and 4% fat.
By permission, courtesy of Mike Anderson, "The RAVE Diet & Lifestyle," www.RaveDiet.com, March 2009, page 142.

(cont. Aztec Salad)….Ingredients List: 3 cups black beans, 2 diced tomatoes, 2 minced garlic cloves, 1 juiced lemon, 10-ounces corn, ¾ cup fresh chopped …cilantro, ½ cup chopped onion, 1 diced/seeded green bell pepper, 1 diced/seeded yellow or red bell pepper, 2 tbsp rice vinegar, 2 tbsp apple cider vinegar, 2 tsp ground cumin, 1 tsp coriander, ½ tsp cayenne pepper.

Directions: In a large bowl, combine beans, corn, onion, bell peppers tomatoes, and cilantro. In a small bowl, whisk together vinegars, lemon juice, garlic, cumin coriander, and cayenne pepper. Pour over salad and mix.

Recipe #14 Broccoli Salad
This recipe makes 4 servings, contains 2 ½ grams fiber & 30 calories per serving as 67% carbohydrate, 26% protein, and 7% fat.
By permission, courtesy of Mike Anderson, "The RAVE Diet & Lifestyle," www.RaveDiet.com, March 2009, page 144.
Ingredients List: 1 bunch broccoli, 2 garlic minced cloves, 1/2 cup sliced onion, ½ cup rice vinegar, 1 tbsp vegetable broth, ½ tsp red pepper flakes/cayenne pepper ground.
Directions: Cut or brake broccoli into small florets. Transfer to a salad bowl. Add remaining ingredients and toss to mix. Chill 20 minutes tossing once or twice before serving.

Recipe #15 Crunchy Salad
This recipe makes 6 servings, contains 3 grams fiber & 46 calories per serving as 85% carbohydrate, 10% protein, and 5% fat.
By permission, courtesy of Mike Anderson, "The RAVE Diet & Lifestyle," www.RaveDiet.com, March 2009, page 145.

(cont. Recipe #15 Crunchy Salad)…
Ingredients List: 15 ounces diced beets, 2 diced carrots, 1 diced jicama, 3 tbsp lemon juice, 2 tbsp rice vinegar, 2 tsp stone ground mustard, ½ tsp dried dill weed.
Directions: Place diced beets, jicama, and carrots into a large salad bowl. In a small bowl, mix lemon juice, vinegar, mustard, and dill; pour over salad into the large salad bowl. Toss to mix and serve of chill before serving.

Recipe #16 Cucumber Arame-Wakame Salad
This recipe makes 4 servings, contains 2 grams fiber & 16 calories per serving as 69% carbohydrate, 31% protein, and 0% fat.
By permission, courtesy of Mike Anderson, "The RAVE Diet & Lifestyle," www.RaveDiet.com, March 2009, page 145. Ingredients List: 1 cucumber, 1 cup arame or 1 cup wakame, 1 cup water, 2 tbsp lemon juice, 2 tbsp water, 1 tbsp rice vinegar, 1 tsp low-sodium Tamari soy sauce.
Directions: Peel and halve cucumber lengthwise. Transfer to a bowl and let stand for 15 minutes. Drain thoroughly. Meanwhile soak the arame/wakame seaweeds in 1 cup of water until soft for 10-15 minutes. Mix together lemon juice, Tamari, vinegar and 2 tbsp water to make dressing. Drain excess water from arame/wakame then combine with cucumber and dressing.

Recipe #17 Pasta Salad
This recipe makes 8 servings, contains 6 grams fiber & 79 calories per serving as 74% carbohydrate, 18% protein, and 8% fat.
By permission, courtesy of Mike Anderson, "The RAVE Diet & Lifestyle," www.RaveDiet.com, March 2009, page 148.

(cont. Recipe #17 Pasta Salad)
Ingredients List: 12 ounces pasta shells, 2 cups/16 ounces artichoke hearts, 3 cups button mushrooms, 1 garlic clove, 1 diced bell pepper, ½ cup chopped green onions, 1/3 cup rice vinegar, ¼ cup cider vinegar, 3 tbsp water, 3 tbsp chopped parsley, 2 tbsp lemon juice, 2 tbsp Dijon mustard, ½ tsp basil, ½ tsp oregano, ¼ tsp black pepper.
Directions: Cook pasta until tender. Rinse and drain, place in large salad bowl. Add artichoke hearts and mushrooms. In a blender, combine vinegars, lemon juice, mustard, ¼ cup green onions, garlic, and seasonings, with 3 tbsp water. Process until smooth. Pour over pasta, and allow to marinate until cool. Add the remaining green onions, parsley, bell pepper, and gently toss to mix.

Recipe #18 Rice Salad
This recipe makes 16 servings, containing 3 grams fiber in each 74 calorie serving as 82% carbohydrate, 11% protein, and 7% fat.
By permission, courtesy of Mike Anderson, "The RAVE Diet & Lifestyle," www.RaveDiet.com, March 2009, page 148.
Ingredients List: 3 cups brown rice, 3 diced roma tomatoes, 1 chopped red/yellow pepper, 1 chopped cucumber, 1 cup chopped raw green beans, ½ cup sliced basil leaves, ½ cup rice vinegar, 1 tbsp mustard, ½ tsp dried parsley flakes, ½ tsp Italian seasoning, 1 juiced lemon.
Directions: In bowl, mix together rice, pepper, green beans, cucumber, tomatoes, and basil. Stir together mustard, rice vinegar, lemon juice, and parsley. Pour over salad and toss to mix. Toss and serve.

Recipe #19 Stuffed Tomato Salad

This recipe makes 5 servings, contains 16 grams fiber & 323 calories per serving as 65% carbohydrate, 20% protein, and 14% fat.

By permission, courtesy of Mike Anderson, The RAVE Diet & Lifestyle, www.RaveDiet.com, March 2009, page 150.

Ingredients List: 5 large ripe tomatoes, 2 cups garbanzo beans, 1 stalk chopped celery.

Directions: Scoop out tomatoes, saving pulp for a sauce. Fill tomatoes with beans and celery. Season with pepper to taste, and garnish with spinach.

Recipe #20 Three-Bean Salad

This recipe makes 4 servings, contains 31 grams fiber in each 589-calories per serving as 68% carbohydrate, 22% protein, and 10% fat.

By permission, courtesy of Mike Anderson, "The RAVE Diet & Lifestyle," www.RaveDiet.com, March 2009, page 151.

Ingredients List: 2 cups kidney beans, 2 cups garbanzo beans, 2 cups lima beans 1 cup chopped onion, ½ cup chopped green pepper, 4 tsp vegetable broth.

Directions: Toss ingredients together. Serve hot or cold with bread or serve cold only as a salad seasoned with a few drops of lemon juice.

Recipe #21 Chickpea Pita Pocket Sandwich

This recipe makes 4 servings, containing 7 grams fiber with each 273-calorie serving as 82% carbohydrate, 12% protein, and 6% fat.

By permission, courtesy of Mike Anderson, "The RAVE Diet & Lifestyle," www.RaveDiet.com, March 2009, page 196.

(cont. Recipe #21 Chickpea Pita Pocket Sandwich)
Ingredients List: 4 whole wheat pitas, 16 ounces mashed chickpeas, 1/3 cup chopped celery, 1 tbl minced onion, 1 tbsp dill pickle relish, 2 tbsp mustard, ¼ tsp garlic powder, 1 sliced tomato, 1 cup diced spinach.
Directions: Place chickpeas, celery onion, relish, mustard, and garlic powder in a bowl and mix well. Cut pitas in half to open pockets; fill (each pita pocket with 1/4th of the spread, then top with tomato slices and diced spinach.

Recipe #22 Portobello Sandwich
This recipe makes 4 sandwiches containing 5 grams fiber per 256 calorie per sandwich as 69% carbohydrate, 24% protein, and 6% fat.
By permission, courtesy of Mike Anderson, "The RAVE Diet & Lifestyle," www.RaveDiet.com, March 2009, page 197.
Ingredients List: 4 large Portobello mushrooms, 4 whole wheat buns, 1 cup red wine vinegar, 1 cup vegetable broth, 1 cup low-sodium Tamari soy sauce, 1 diced onion.
Directions: Mix vinegar, vegetable broth, and Tamari in blender then pour over mushrooms and allow to sit overnight. Add to mushrooms diced or sliced onion and tomato topping to each sandwich bun.

Recipe #23 Lentil Burger
This recipe makes 8 burgers, containing 3 grams fiber with each 95-calorie burger as 87 % carbohydrate, 11% protein, and 2% fat.
By permission, courtesy of Mike Anderson, "The RAVE Diet & Lifestyle," www.RaveDiet.com, March 2009, page 178.

(cont. Recipe #23 Lentil Burger)…Ingredients List: 1-diced onion, ½ cup short-grain brown rice, ½ cup lentils, 2 cups water, 1 carrot, 1 celery stalk, 2-tsp stone ground mustard, 1 tsp garlic powder, pureed fruit of choice for skillet.

Directions: In a medium-size saucepan, combine onion, rice, lentils, and water. Bring to slow simmer, then cover and cook for 50 minutes, or until rice & lentils are tender and all the water has been absorbed. Chop carrot and celery until fine, and add them and all ingredients into the hot lentil mix; stir this mix then chill completely. Form chilled mix into 2-3 inch patties. Lightly coat skillet with pureed fruits such as banana, apricot, or peach.

Recipe #24 Vegetarian Chili

This recipe makes 4 servings, containing 19 grams fiber in each 344 calorie serving as 71% carbohydrate, 21% protein, and 8% fat.

By permission, courtesy of Mike Anderson, "The RAVE Diet & Lifestyle," www.RaveDiet.com, March 2009, page 180.

Ingredients List: 4 cups pinto beans, 3 minced jalapeno peppers, 1 chopped onion, 1 diced bell pepper, 1 cup diced tomatoes, 2 cups vegetable broth, ¼ cup chopped cilantro, 2 tsp chili powder, 1 tbsp chopped garlic, 1 tsp ground cumin, 1 tsp oregano, 2 tsp corn meal.

(cont. Recipe #24 Vegetarian Chili)...Directions: In oven, sauté onion, bell pepper, and garlic in a small portion vegetable broth until onion is translucent. Add jalapeno peppers, cumin, chili powder, and oregano. Stir until the spices are fragrant. Add the beans, chopped tomatoes, all but 3 tablespoons of vegetable broth and cilantro. Set the remaining vegetable broth aside. Bring the chili to a boil. Reduce the heat and simmer, uncovered, for 10 minutes. Place the corn meal in a small bowl. Mix in the reserved vegetable broth, stirring to make a smooth mixture. While stirring the chili, blend in the corn meal and mix. Continue simmering the chili 10 minutes. Put in refrigerator for 2-hours before serving (Chilling enhances the flavor remarkably).

Recipe #25 Vegetarian Falafel

This recipe makes 8 servings, containing 6 grams fiber in each 200 calorie serving as 55% carbohydrate, 18% protein, and 27% fat.

By permission, courtesy of Mike Anderson, "The RAVE Diet & Lifestyle," www.RaveDiet.com, March 2009, page 183.

Ingredients List: 33 ounces chick peas (garbanzo beans), 6 green chopped green onions, 4 minced garlic cloves, 1/3 cup whole wheat flour, ¼ cup parsley, ¼ cup water, 1 tbsp lemon juice, 1 tsp turmeric.

Directions: Mix everything but flour in food processor or mash it completely. Add flour and stir till well mixed. Form into small patties and bake at 375, turn until both sides are crispy, wrap in spinach leaves. This Falafel is dipped into favorite sauce.

Recipe #26 Fruit Dessert (Lower Calorie Version of Fruit Cobbler)

(cont. Recipe #26 Fruit Dessert (Lower Calorie Version of Fruit Cobbler)This recipe makes 8 servings, containing 5 grams fiber with each 229 calorie serving as 69% carbohydrate, 3% protein, and 29% fat.

By permission, courtesy of Celia Misner, Spokane, Washington.

(Ingredients List: 16 ounces Blueberries, 12 ounces blackberries, 4 peaches, 1 can peach pie filling, 1-8" x 11" pyrex pan pie crust, ¼ cup brown sugar (or Xylitol Sweetening crystals), ½ cup rolled oats, 1 tbsp cinnamon.

 (Lower Calorie Version of Fruit Cobbler)

Directions: Dump pie filling into a large 2 quart mixing bowl. Cover with sliced peaches, leave skins on. Lightly sprinkle with brown sugar and allow a few minutes to "soak in" to the fruit. Add a layer of blueberries and a layer of blackberries. Stir gently to avoid tearing the fruit. Cut piecrust to fit on an 8" x 11" pyrex glass baking dish. Use fork to put small punctures into the crust. Pour in fruit mixture. Sprinkle uncooked rolled oats and cinnamon over the fruit mixture (there is no need for a high fat shortening or butter in this recipe. Cover the dish with a sheet of heavy-duty aluminum foil and bake at 350 degrees for 45 minutes. (Warning juices from dish can leak into oven; a drip pan beneath is recommended. Cool and cut into squares.

Recipe #27 Cheese Sauce Topping

This recipe makes 4-6 servings, containing 5-8 grams fiber in each 90-130 calorie serving as 60% carbohydrate, 31% protein, and 9% fat. By permission, courtesy of Mike Anderson, "The RAVE Diet & Lifestyle," www.RaveDiet.com, March 2009, page 208.

(cont. Recipe #27 Cheese Sauce Topping)…Ingredients List: 2 cups water, ½ cup nutritional yeast flakes, ½ cup whole-wheat flour, ½ tsp garlic powder, ¼ cup vegetable broth, 1 tsp mustard.

Directions: In a 2-quart saucepan, mix together nutritional yeast flakes, flour and garlic powder, then add 2 cups water. Cook over medium heat, whisking until it thickens and bubbles. Cook 30 seconds more, then remove from heat and whisk in vegetable broth and mustard. Sauce will thicken as it cools but will thin when heated. Good for a casserole, a topping for lasagna, or pan of enchiladas.

Recipe #28 Banana Cake
This recipe makes 8 servings, containing 5 grams fiber in each 212 calorie serving as 88% carbohydrate, 8% protein, and 3% fat.

By permission, courtesy of Mike Anderson, "The RAVE Diet & Lifestyle," www.RaveDiet.com, March 2009, page 216.

Ingredients List: 4 ripe bananas, 2 cups whole wheat pastry flour, 1 ½ tsp baking soda, ½ cup maple syrup, 1/3 cup applesauce, ¼ cup water, 1 tsp vanilla extract.

Directions: Preheat oven to 350. Mix flour, baking soda in a bowl. In a large bowl, beat maple syrup and applesauce together. Add bananas and mash them. Stir in water and vanilla and mix thoroughly and add flour mixture and stir to mix. Spread in a 9-inch baking pan. Bake for 45-50 minutes, or until a toothpick inserted into the center comes out clean.

Recipe #29 Sweet Potato Pudding
This recipe makes 4 servings, containing 1 gram fiber, in each 178 calorie serving) as 89% carbohydrate, 8% protein, and 3% fat.

(cont. Recipe #29 Sweet Potato Pudding) By permission, courtesy of Mike Anderson, "The RAVE Diet & Lifestyle," www.RaveDiet.com, March 2009, page 223. Ingredients List: 2 cups cooked sweet potato or yam, 1-cup water, 2/3 cup rolled oats, 2 tbsp maple syrup, and ¼ tsp cinnamon.
Directions: Combine all ingredients in blender and blend to smooth texture. Chill before serving.

Recipe #30 Gingerbread Cookies
This recipe makes 48 cookies, containing 1-gram fiber and 33 calories in each cookie as 88% carbohydrate, 9% protein, and 3% fat.
By permission, courtesy of Mike Anderson, "The RAVE Diet & Lifestyle," www.RaveDiet.com, March 2009, page 218.
Ingredients List: 2 ¼ cups whole wheat pastry flour, 1/3 cup molasses, 1/3 cup water, ½ cup maple syrup, 1 ½ tsp baking soda, 1 tsp ground ginger, 1 tsp cinnamon.
Directions: Mix the maple syrup, ginger, cinnamon and baking soda in a large bowl. Add the molasses and water and mix well. Add 1 cup of flour and mix well. Mix in enough of the remaining flour to make very stiff dough. Preheat oven to 275. Dust up to 3 baking sheets with flour. On a floured surface, roll a portion of the dough with a flour-dusted rolling pin to a very fine thickness, about 1/16th inch thickness. Cut the dough into shapes with a flour dusted cookie cutter or flour-dusted knife. Transfer the cookies to the baking sheets.
Bake until the edges are dry and the centers give when slightly pressed or about 20 minutes. Allow cooling on baking sheet for 5 minutes, and then transferring with a spatula to a wire rack to cool. Once cooled, store in an airtight container.

Recipe #31 Fifteen 15 Bean Soup

This recipe makes 12 servings, containing 4 grams fiber in each 93 calorie serving as 59% carbohydrate, 36% protein, and 5% fat.

By permission, courtesy of Celia Misner, Spokane, Washington.

Ingredients List: 16 ounces Hurst's HamBeens brand 15 Bean Soup ("15 Bean Soup" contains the following: northern beans, pinto beans, large lima beans, blackeye, garbanzo, baby lima beans, green split, kidney, cranberry beans, small white beans, pink beans, small red beans, yellow split, lentil, navy, white kidney, & black bean.), ½ red onion, ½ chopped green or yellow bell pepper, 6 chopped button or enoki or shitake mushrooms (choice left to individual preference), 1 tbsp Johnny's Seasoning Salt, 2 tbsp sea salt, 1 tbsp black pepper, 3-4 quarts distilled water, ½ package Soy Crumbles.

Directions: Rinse beans and soak overnight in enough water to cover thoroughly. Next day put all ingredients into a slow cooker crock-pot and cook on high for 4 hours. Turn on "low" and continue cooking until beans are soft. Serve with warm bread or rolls.

Recipe #32 Ginger Ale

This recipe makes 1 serving 16 fluid ounces, contains 1-gram fiber, 118 calories per serving as 96% carbohydrate, 3% protein, and 1% fat.

By permission, courtesy of Brendan Brazier, "THRIVE, The Vegan Nutrition Guide to Optimal Performance in Sports and Life," De Capo Press, 2008, page 269.

Ingredients List: 2 cups water, 1 lemon, 1 tbsp agave nectar, ½ tbsp fresh ginger, sea salt to taste (cont. Recipe #32 Ginger Ale)…Directions: Squeeze the juice of a lemon into a blender. Add water, agave nectar, ginger, and sea salt; blend and may store in refrigerator up to 2 weeks.

Recipe #33 Sweet Potato Premiere
This recipe makes 1-2 servings, contains 8 grams fiber in each 354 calorie serving as 91% carbohydrate, 6% protein, and 3% fat. This makes a delicious dessert that may be eaten alone for breakfast.
Ingredients List: 1 large sweet potato, 2-fluid ounces water, 2 ounces steel cut oats (or rolled oats), 1-ounce psyllium husk powder, 1-ounce xylitol, 1 tsp ground cinnamon, ¼ cup raisins
Directions: Cook sweet potato in oven 350 degrees 45 minutes or until softened well. Mix and in 2-fluid ounces warm water the remaining ingredients steel cut oats (or rolled oats), psyllium husk powder, xylitol, ground cinnamon, and raisins to make a paste. Stir, mix, and mash paste into the whole baked sweet potato.

CHAPTER XII Healthy Meal - Frequently Asked Questions

➢ *What macronutrient-percents of carbohydrate, protein, and fat should I eat?* The goal of a heart healthy plant foods diet is 75%+ Carbohydrate, 5-10% Protein [+/- 5%], and no more than 10% Fat (No Oils, No Nuts, No Seeds!)

➢ *What do I eat in place of fats, butters, margarines and oils?* Fat Substitutes are replaced by pureed fruits, applesauce, vegetable stock, and vinegars or cooking with pureed baby fruits will replace the oils-fats tastes and cravings.

➢ *What do I eat for "sweets" craving in place of highly processed sugary sweets?* Each of the following contains a good nutrient profile, but these should not be excessively consumed since most have copious amounts of natural simple sugar: Agave Nectar, Barley Malt, Maple Sugar, Black Strap Molasses, Sorghum Syrup, and dried fruits. The following spices produce a "Sweet" taste sensation: Anise, Cardamon, Cinnamon, Fenugreek, Paprika, and Vanilla.

➢ *What should I eat in terms of dietary fiber for colon health?* This is a very, very important question. While most nutritionists are not agreed on whether soluble or insoluble fiber is best for health, they are agreed on the need to consume at least 30-grams total fiber in foods per day. Soluble fiber slows stomach emptying while insoluble fiber hastens it. Both forms of fiber increase the rate of bowel transit time to emptying food wastes.

This is important because bulk fiber in the bowel removes wastes on bowel walls and some of the nutrients in the food that can raise blood fats or sugars too high too fast. Americans typically consume only 11-14 grams fiber per day…way too little to impact healthy gastric function. While most of the responsible favorable research in this arena has been performed on soluble fiber, there is enough research on insoluble fiber to recommend 50% soluble and 50% insoluble fiber in the ideal menu. Soluble fiber dissolves in water and forms a gel-like paste. It has a remarkable cholesterol-lowering effect. Soluble fiber is found in legumes, vegetables, fruits, and whole grains such as peas, beans, potatoes, sweet potatoes, onions, artichokes, broccoli, carrots barley, rye, oats, apples, pears, plums, berries, bananas contain soluble fiber. Insoluble fiber does not dissolve in water and it is found skins of fruits, all vegetables, and all whole grains. Insoluble fibers prevent constipation by absorbing water into the stools, making them soft and bulky, quenching appetite, and increasing bowel transit time.

Many of the plant foods that have soluble fiber also have insoluble fiber. Eating 50% each both soluble-insoluble fiber foods decreases the absorption of fat and sugars reducing absorption of calories. This maintains a normal blood-sugar level and reduces cholesterol. A high fiber intake increases peristalsis moving toxic waste through the intestines quickly. While the daily recommended value total fiber is only 30 grams per day, I have observed healthy individuals consume above 60 grams fiber per day. Persons getting adequate calories from a whole plant food lifestyle are most likely receiving adequate amounts of both soluble and insoluble fiber.

- *What do I need eat in terms of raw plant foods versus cooked plant foods?* When a plant food is cooked, many of its nutrient effects are lost. I recommend consuming as many whole plant foods as possible raw. Most persons consuming a plant food diet can consume 50% whole plant foods raw and 50% of their foods cooked. Keep in mind; most plant foods can be consumed raw without cooking or altering nutrient content. Beans are an exception to eating in raw form once they become hard; they need to be prepared. Soaking beans until they are soft helps break down the complex carbohydrates (oligiosaccharides) beans contain. Soaking will reduce flatulence and improve digestion. A well-soaked dry bean increases to twice its original size and when cut open, it will be soft inside. Always throw away water used for soaking since some beans release toxic substances and gas-forming oligiosaccharides they contain. Soaking beans in the refrigerator for 8-10 hours is recommended. Cooking beans may or may not be preferred, since cooking will denature and reduce further the protein content. Cooking is optional, while making sure the bean is completely soft after soaking is required. There is slightly more protein and gas-forming oligiosaccharides in a soaked bean compared to a soaked and cooked bean.
- *What condiments, sauces, flavorings are safe to add to a whole plant food menu?* A1 Steak Sauce, Tobasco Sauce, Teriyaki Sauce, Tomato Ketchup, Salsa, Dijon Mustard, Tamari Sauce, Bragg Liquid Aminos; chose only low-sodium/low-fat mustards, ketchups, and tomato sauces.

➢ *What ingredients additives should be avoided?* Avoid all hydrogenated oils, alum, artificial colorings, BHT, Calcium propionate, casein, casinogen, diglycerides, monoglycerides, gelatin, collagen, glycerin, glycerides, hydrolysates, anything hydrolyzed or hydrogenated, lactic acid, lactose, lactulose, lard, mono-glycerides, mono-diglycerides, monosodium glutamate MSG, mycoprotein, palmitate, polysorbates, rennet, rennin sodium caseinate, sodium nitrate, sugars, sulfites, vegetable oils, and whey. This is not a complete list. One rule of thumb is if an ingredient is hard to pronounce, it may not be advisable to consume it.

➢ *What fruits should be avoided?* Fruits have stickers indicating how they were grown; any sticker that has #4011 is a conventionally grown, pesticide treated fruit, #84011 is a genetically engineered fruit. Avoid these.

➢ *What fruits are best to eat?* Fruits have stickers indicating how they were grown; any sticker that has #94011 is organic grown.

Phytonutrition: Finding Fitness For Life! – 2nd Edition
This book argues favorably for changing your diet to eating only whole plant foods. The biggest obstacle to such change is individual habitual learned appetite shaped by both nature and nurture. We possess a nature that is born attracted to calorie-dense foods. Animal food calories are denser than plant foods. Western nations nurture and educate their populace to buy animal source foods designed to attract taste but block satiated state. In nations where animal source calories have replaced whole plant foods, the onset of cardiovascular disease, diabetes, cancer, and autoimmune diseases have risen dramatically. In nations where whole plant foods predominate, the rate of cardiovascular disease, diabetes, cancer, and autoimmune diseases is significantly less. Whole plant food nutrition advocates such as Dr. T. Colin Campbell, Dr. Joel Fuhrman, Dr. Caldwell Esselstyn Jr., Dr. John Mcdougall, and Mike Anderson, report patients who completely resolved very serious health problems by adopting the whole plant foods lifestyle and eliminating all animal source foods from their diet. This book shows how and what foods provide the nutrients that produce energy and health and dietary associations with compromised health and premature death. The proof is determined by a 90-days trial test, which is confirmed by weight loss, lower body mass index, and lower cholesterol. The author guarantees results. **The decision now belongs to you...**

9 781304 866332